Understanding health services

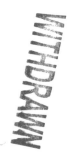

Nick Black and Reinhold Gruen

Understanding Public Health

Series editors: Nick Black and Rosalind Raine, London School of Hygiene & Tropical Medicine

Throughout the world, recognition of the importance of public health to sustainable, safe and healthy societies is growing. The achievements of public health in nineteenth-century Europe were for much of the twentieth century overshadowed by advances in personal care, in particular in hospital care. Now, with the dawning of a new century, there is increasing understanding of the inevitable limits of individual health care and of the need to complement such services with effective public health strategies. Major improvements in people's health will come from controlling communicable diseases, eradicating environmental hazards, improving people's diets and enhancing the availability and quality of effective health care. To achieve this, every country needs a cadre of knowledgeable public health practitioners with social, political and organizational skills to lead and bring about changes at international, national and local levels.

This is one of a series of 20 books that provides a foundation for those wishing to join in and contribute to the twenty-first-century regeneration of public health, helping to put the concerns and perspectives of public health at the heart of policy-making and service provision. While each book stands alone, together they provide a comprehensive account of the three main aims of public health: protecting the public from environmental hazards, improving the health of the public and ensuring high quality health services are available to all. Some of the books focus on methods, others on key topics. They have been written by staff at the London School of Hygiene & Tropical Medicine with considerable experience of teaching public health to students from low, middle and high income countries. Much of the material has been developed and tested with postgraduate students both in face-to-face teaching and through distance learning.

The books are designed for self-directed learning. Each chapter has explicit learning objectives, key terms are highlighted and the text contains many activities to enable the reader to test their own understanding of the ideas and material covered. Written in a clear and accessible style, the series will be essential reading for students taking postgraduate courses in public health and will also be of interest to public health practitioners and policy-makers.

Titles in the series

Analytical models for decision making: Colin Sanderson and Reinhold Gruen
Controlling communicable disease: Norman Noah
Economic analysis for management and policy: Stephen Jan, Lilani Kumaranayake,
    Jenny Roberts, Kara Hanson and Kate Archibald
Economic evaluation: Julia Fox-Rushby and John Cairns (eds)
Environmental epidemiology: Paul Wilkinson (ed)
Environment, health and sustainable development: Megan Landon
Environmental health policy: David Ball
Financial management in health services: Reinhold Gruen and Anne Howarth
Global change and health: Kelley Lee and Jeff Collin (eds)
Health care evaluation: Sarah Smith, Don Sinclair, Rosalind Raine and Barnaby Reeves
Health promotion practice: Maggie Davies, Wendy Macdowall and Chris Bonell (eds)
Health promotion theory: Maggie Davies and Wendy Macdowall (eds)
Introduction to epidemiology: Lucianne Bailey, Katerina Vardulaki, Julia Langham and
    Daniel Chandramohan
Introduction to health economics: David Wonderling, Reinhold Gruen and Nick Black
Issues in public health: Joceline Pomerleau and Martin McKee (eds)
Making health policy: Kent Buse, Nicholas Mays and Gill Walt
Managing health services: Nick Goodwin, Reinhold Gruen and Valerie Iles
Medical anthropology: Robert Pool and Wenzel Geissler
Principles of social research: Judith Green and John Browne (eds)
Understanding health services: Nick Black and Reinhold Gruen

Understanding health services

Nick Black and Reinhold Gruen

Open University Press

Open University Press
McGraw-Hill Education
McGraw-Hill House
Shoppenhangers Road
Maidenhead
Berkshire
England
SL6 2QL

email: enquiries@openup.co.uk
world wide web: www.openup.co.uk

and Two Penn Plaza, New York, NY 10121-2289, USA

First published 2005

A catalogue record of this book is available from the British Library

ISBN-10: 0 335 21838 5
ISBN-13: 978 0335 21838 7

Library of Congress Cataloging-in-Publication Data
CIP data applied for

Typeset by RefineCatch Limited, Bungay, Suffolk
Printed in the UK by Bell & Bain Ltd, Glasgow

Contents

Acknowledgements

Open University Press and the London School of Hygiene and Tropical Medicine have made every effort to obtain permission from copyright holders to reproduce material in this book and to acknowledge these sources correctly. Any omissions brought to our attention will be remedied in future editions.

We would like to express our grateful thanks to the following copyright holders for granting permission to reproduce material in this book.

p. 93   Reprinted with permission from Audit Commission (2001). Acute hospital portfolio. Review of national findings. Day Surgery. London: Audit Commission for England and Wales.

p. 106–7   Reprinted from Social Science and Medicine, Vol 48, M Bernhart, IGP Wiadnyana, H Wihardjo, I Pohan, 'Patient satisfaction in developing countries', pp989–996, copyright (1999), with permission from Elsevier.

p. 16–18   Reprinted with permission from Elsevier (The Lancet, 1997, Vol 349, No. 9068, Black, pp 1834–1835).

p. 98–101   Journal of Epidemiology and Community Health, 1995, 49: 408–412, reproduced with permission from the BMJ Publishing Group.

p. 191–93   Reprinted with permission from Buchan J, Dal Poz MR (2002). Skill mix in the health care workforce: reviewing the evidence. Bulletin of the WHO 80:575–80.

p. 110–12   Reprinted with permission from Byrne PS, Long BEL (1976). Doctors talking to patients: a study of the verbal behaviour of GPs consulting in their surgeries, HMSO, London. Crown copyright material is reproduced with the permission of the Controller of HMSO and the Queen's Printer for Scotland.

p. 136–38   Reproduced from the Journal of Health Services Research & Policy 1997; 2(1): 3–4 with the permission of the Royal Society of Medicine Press, London.

p. 210–11   Reproduced from the Journal of Health Services Research & Policy 1999; 4(4): 193–194 with the permission of the Royal Society of Medicine Press, London.

p. 228–30   W de Geyndt, Improving the quality of health care in Latin America, International Journal for Quality in Health Care, 2001, 13(2), 85–87, by permission of Oxford University Press.

p. 196–98   Reproduced from the Journal of Health Services Research & Policy 2002; 7(1): 1–2 with the permission of the Royal Society of Medicine Press, London.

p. 179   Reprinted with permission from the World Health Organization from A Y Ellencweig, 1992, Analysing Health Systems, A Modular approach.

p. 44   Reprinted from Fink-Anthe C (1992). Kulturell beeinflußte Therapiegewohnheiten: Bedeutung für den europäischen Markt. Deutsche Apotheker Zeitung 29:1534–39.

p. 155–59   Frenk J and Donabedian A, State intervention in medical care: types, trends and variables, Health Policy and Planning, 1987, 2(1), 17–31, by permission of Oxford University Press.

p. 170–71   Reprinted by permission of Oxford University Press. Green A (1999). An introduction to health planning in developing countries (2nd ed). Oxford: Oxford University Press.

p. 214–16   Reproduced from the Journal of Health Services Research & Policy 1998; 3(2): 67–69 with the permission of the Royal Society of Medicine Press, London.

p. 37–39   Reproduced from King L (1954) What is disease? Philosophy of Science 1:193–203, with permission from the University of Chicago.

p. 59–61 Last M (1996). The professionalisation of indigenous healers, in Sergent C, Johnson T (eds) Medical anthropology: contemporary theory and method. Westport: Praeger. Reproduced with permission of Greenwood Publishing Group, Inc., Westport, CT.

p. 120–23 Reproduced from the Journal of Health Services Research & Policy 1997; 2(2): 103–111 with the permission of the Royal Society of Medicine Press, London.

p. 218–19 Reproduced from the Journal of Health Services Research & Policy 2000; 5(1): 1–2 with the permission of the Royal Society of Medicine Press, London.

p. 70–73 Reproduced from Health Economics: An international perspective, McPake B, Kumaranayake L, Normand C, 2002, London: Routledge, with permission of the Taylor and Francis Group.

p. 180–81 Reproduced with permission Healthlink Worldwide from McPake, B (1994), 'Initiative for Change', in Health Action, Issue 9, pp7, Healthlink Worldwide, London.

p. 145–51 Mills AJ, Ransom K (2001). The design of health systems, in Merson MH, Black RE, Mills AJ (eds) International public health, diseases, programs, systems and policies. Jones and Bartlett Publishers, Sudbury, MA. *www.jbpub.com.* Reprinted with permission.

p. 26–29 Reprinted from Msiska R, Nangawe E, Mulenga D, Sichone M, Kamanga J, Kwapa P (1997). Understanding lay perspectives: care options for STD treatment in Lusaka, Zambia. Health Policy & Planning 12:248–252, by permission of Oxford University Press.

p. 42–43 Excerpt adapted from MEDICINE & CULTURE by Lynn Payer. Copyright © 1988 by Lynn Payer. Reprinted by permission of Henry Holt and Company, LLC.

p. 97 Reprinted from Polder JJ, Bonneaux L, Meeding WJ, van der Maas PJ (2002). Age-specific increases in health care costs. European Journal of Public Health 12:58, by permission of Oxford University Press.

p. 185–86 Reproduced from Poore P (2004). The Global Fund to fight Aids, Tuberculosis and Malaria (GFATM). Health Policy & Planning 19:52–3, by permission of Oxford University Press.

p. 13–14 Reproduced from Relman AS (1988). Assessment and accountability. The third revolution in medical care. New England Journal of Medicine 319:1220–2, with permission from Massachusetts Medical Society. Adapted with permission from MMS.

p. 84–86 Reproduced from Stevens A, Gabbay J (1991). Needs assessment needs assessment . . . Health Trends 23:20–3. Crown copyright material is reproduced with the permission of the Controller of HMSO and the Queen's Printer for Scotland.

p. 56–58 Reproduced from Strong PM, Robinson J (1990). The NHS. Under new management. Milton Keynes: Open University Press, with kind permission of the Open University Press/McGraw-Hill Publishing Company.

p. 174–77 Reprinted from Walsh JA, Warren KS (1980). Selective primary health care: an interim strategy for disease control in developing countries. Social Science & Medicine 14C:145–63, with permission from Elsevier.

p. 182–83 'Box 1: Investing in Health', from WORLD DEVELOPMENT REPORT 1993 by World Bank, copyright © 1993 by The International Bank for Reconstruction and Development/The World Bank. Used by permission of Oxford University Press, Inc.

p. 173 'Box 6.2: Community health workers', from WORLD DEVELOPMENT REPORT 1993 by World Bank, copyright © 1993 by The International Bank for Reconstruction and Development/The World Bank. Used by permission of Oxford University Press, Inc.

Overview of the book

Introduction

Public health is as much concerned with the provision and performance of health services as with activities to promote health and prevent disease. While impossible to quantify accurately, it seems that the improvements in the health of the public over the past century may be equally due to three factors: personal health care (the treatment of disease); disease prevention (such as immunization and changes in personal behaviour); and social policies (such as policies to improve nutrition and housing).

No single discipline can provide a full account of how and why health care is the way it is. This book provides you with a series of conceptual frameworks which help to understand the apparent complexity that confronts the inexperienced observer. It demonstrates the need for a multidisciplinary approach to understanding health services and the contributions that medicine, sociology, economics, history and epidemiology make. It also shows how it is necessary to consider health care at three key levels: the micro level of the individual patient and their experiences; the meso level of how health care organizations such as health centres and hospitals work; and the macro level of regional and national institutions such as governments and health insurance bodies.

Many of the themes raised in this book are developed in greater depth in companion volumes. Our aim here is to provide an overview that will help you place specific aspects of health services in a wider context.

You will have adopted your own view on health services, based on your professional background and experience. This view will help you as you work through the book. However, no specialist knowledge is required. The approach taken will broaden your view on health services and explain why health systems are the way they are.

The concepts presented rarely take the form of exact definitions, such as you come across in statistics and epidemiology or when studying physical sciences. Rather they should help you interpret complex issues and form your own perspective on health services.

Why study health services?

Before embarking, it is worth considering why health services should be a subject of study. There are several reasons (and you may have others):

1 Health is of primary importance to most people.
2 Health services contribute to maintaining and improving people's health.

3 There is uncertainty as to the effectiveness, humanity, equity and efficiency of many interventions.
4 There is a need to make health care professionals and services more accountable to the public.
5 Expenditure on health care represents a large and growing proportion of national budgets.
6 Health services are a major employer.
7 The medical-industrial complex that supplies health services is a major power and influence on national governments and international health organizations.

Structure of the book

This book follows the conceptual outline of the 'health services' unit at the London School of Hygiene & Tropical Medicine. It is based on the materials presented in the lectures and seminars of the taught course, which have been adapted for distance learning.

The book is structured around a simple conceptual framework. It starts by looking at the inputs to health services, goes on to consider the processes of care, and then discusses the outcomes. But a health system is more than just its parts. So you then consider the way the components are organized. Finally, you consider how the quality of health care can be assessed and improved.

The six sections, and the 20 chapters within them, are shown on the book's contents page. Each chapter includes:

- an overview
- a list of learning objectives
- a list of key terms
- a range of activities
- feedback on the activities
- a summary.

Although examples and case studies in this book are balanced between low, middle and high income countries, you should be aware that most of the theory on health systems has been derived in high income countries.

The following description of the section and chapter contents will give you an idea of what you will be reading.

Introduction. Chapter 1 explains the rationale for using a systems approach to the analysis of health services, while Chapter 2 considers the principal challenges facing health services. Like most books in this area, you will be reading and learning about formal health care. Despite the huge role of informal or lay care, it has remained little studied. Before proceeding, therefore, in Chapter 3 the contribution of lay care and its relationship to formal care are considered.

Inputs to health care. Chapters 4 and 5 provide a conceptual framework for understanding how medical knowledge shapes a key input, that of patients and their diseases. In Chapter 6 you will consider a second input, that of staff. You will learn what a profession is and examine in particular the relationship between doctors and nurses. Chapter 7 gets you to consider the other essential input, finance. The chapter also leads on to the next section, by describing the basic features of the resource allocation process in countries with publicly funded health services.

Processes of health care. In this section you will focus first on the concepts of need, demand and use. In Chapter 8 you will learn how to conceptualize need for health care and in Chapter 9 you will examine what factors influence utilization of health services. Chapters 10 and 11 take account of the interaction between staff and users of health services. You will first look at users in their role as patients (Chapter 10) and then in their public role as consumers and members of communities (Chapter 11).

Outcomes of health care. The fourth section considers outcomes, how to define and measure them and the contribution both of objective and subjective approaches.

Organization of services. Chapters 13 and 14 will explain the different methods for comparing health systems and deepen the systems approach used in this book. You will address why health systems are as they are, explore different theories of health systems and consider the role of the state in health care. In the next three chapters you will analyse trends in health care reforms. Chapters 15 and 16 look at the organization of health services in low and middle income countries: the concept of primary care, the debate on the modifications of this concept, and international initiatives which have led to a reorganization of health services in the past two decades. Chapter 17 provides an overview of the organizational aspects of recent reforms of health services in high income countries.

Quality improvement. Chapter 18 introduces the dimensions of quality (effectiveness, humanity and equity), the principles of quality improvement, and how criteria of good quality care can be established through reviews of research evidence and the use of consensus development techniques. Chapter 19 describes methods for assessing the performance of health services, and Chapter 20 considers the range of possible interventions to improve quality.

A variety of activities are employed to help your understanding and learning of the topics and ideas covered. These include:

- reflection on your own knowledge and experience
- questions based on reading key articles or relevant research papers
- analyses of quantitative and qualitative data.

Acknowledgements

The authors would like to acknowledge the important contributions made by colleagues who developed the original lectures and teaching material at the LSHTM on which some of the contents are based: Charles Normand (Chapter 7), Judith Green (Chapters 6, 10 and 11), Martin McKee (Chapters 13, 14 and 17) and Ruairi Brugha (Chapters 15 and 16). The authors would also like to acknowledge the contribution of Dr Myfanwy Morgan, King's College London, for reviewing the book and Deirdre Byrne for managing the production of the whole series.

SECTION 1

Introduction

A systems approach to health services

Overview

The approach to analysing health services in this book is based on systems theory. In this brief introductory chapter you will explore the concept of social systems and learn about the essential elements of health care systems.

Learning objectives

After working through this chapter, you will be better able to:

- identify the basic features of a social system
- identify inputs, processes and outcomes in health care systems.

Key terms

Inputs The resources needed by a system.

Outcomes Change in status as a result of the system processes (in the health services context, the change in health status as a result of care).

Outputs A combination of the processes and outcomes that constitute the total production of a system.

Processes The use of resources or the activity within a system.

System A model of a whole entity, reflecting the relationship between its elements at different levels of complexity.

What are health services?

Before studying health care systems, you need to consider which activities are included under the term 'health services'. For the purposes of this book, the full range of activities that are undertaken *primarily* for health reasons are included. Although some of the most dramatic health benefits are the result of wider policies such as those affecting the environment, education, housing and employment, this book is confined to services that are first and foremost undertaken to have a direct effect on people's health. These extend from health promotion and disease prevention, through curative services, to long term care, rehabilitation and even custody.

What is a system?

The term 'system' is in common use – the human body can be seen as a biological system; an engine can be seen as a technical system. But what is meant by 'health system' as opposed to 'health care' or 'health services'? The following activity is designed to allow you to reflect on the basic features of a social system.

 Activity 1.1

Taking the transport system in the town where you live, carry out the following tasks.

1 Write a brief description of its main constituent parts. Think of the difference between the notion of a system and the elements it is made of. You may find it helpful to draw a rough sketch of the system showing the interrelationships between the parts you describe.
2 Make a list of the different aspects of transport you can look at, for example object-ives, means and processes.

 Feedback

Obviously there is a wide range of possible answers. You may distinguish, for example, between *inputs* – cars, boats and aircraft. Or you may look at the *processes* related to traffic, for example how a traffic jam builds up, the financing of public transport, road maintenance or infrastructure planning; or the *objectives* of the transport system, such as increasing mobility or controlling traffic flows.

A system has:

- a purpose or mission
- decision making processes that are themselves systems – these interact so that their effects can be transmitted throughout the system
- resources that can be used by the decision making process
- some guarantee of continuity.

Furthermore,

- its performance can be measured
- it exists in wider systems and/or environments with which it interacts but from which it is separated.

Generally, a social system represents a set of interdependent elements, which can be seen as a purposeful whole. This means that the perception of a single element cannot account for understanding the whole arrangement. For example, the com-bination of different transport subsystems (such as road, water and air transport) increases mobility more than a single element of transport.

Understanding interdependent phenomena as a system lets you understand how things are organized and how the whole responds to change, if one of its parts changes.

A systems approach to health care

There are clearly many different ways of describing a system but, whatever approach you choose, you need to put the elements in a coherent and meaningful order. The way health services are presented in this book is intended to increase your awareness of the results of health care and how these are achieved. Ultimately, the objective of any health system is to improve people's health. Hence a meaningful approach would describe how health care affects health status. The approach followed in this book is:

Inputs → Processes → Outcomes

- *inputs* are the resources needed for health care
- *processes* describe the use of resources or the activity within the system
- *outcome* is change in health status as result of those processes.

 Activity 1.2

Copy and complete the table below by writing down two examples against each heading. An example of each has been provided to get you started.

Table 1.1

Input	1 Medical equipment
	2
	3
Process	1 Referral to specialist
	2
	3
Outcome	1 Survival
	2
	3

 Feedback

This way of looking at health care brings together elements that belong to a variety of categories.

Inputs. Examples include resources such as staff, land, buildings, funds, medical knowledge, drugs and patients. Did you think of human resources? This is the most important input because it is staff who employ (or use) all other resources. You may not have thought of 'patients' as an input, but without them there would be no processes and, as you will see in Chapters 10 and 11, they play key roles in the production of health.

Processes. Processes are activities within the system, for example investigation and treatment of patients or referral of patients between facilities. Did you think of the therapeutic process? The patient–staff interaction is one of the essential processes of care and you will explore it more in detail later in the book.

You may also think of organizational processes, for example drug supplies, electronic transmission of information, rationing of care, ways of raising money for the health sector or paying staff.

Outcomes. These are the results of care, which can be measured in terms of changes in patients' survival or quality of life. But there are many intermediate measures expressing changes in impairment, such as blood sugar levels, body weight or blood pressure, and changes in disability or functional ability, such as mobility or memory. You will explore the definition and use of outcome measures in Chapter 12.

Why outcomes and not outputs?

You may wonder why you don't look at *outputs* as a result of inputs. Economists use the term 'output' to describe the production process, for example the number of cars produced in an automobile factory. By analogy, health economists apply this concept to a combination of processes and outcomes of health services. You will explore the relationship between inputs and outputs, and between outputs and costs in the health economics books in this series. The systems theory approach used here is somewhat different. The focus is on *outcomes* as a result of inputs and processes, and this concept emphasizes the change in health status as a result of care.

Summary

As with other social systems, health services can be seen as a set of interdependent elements that constitute a purposeful whole. In order to describe how health care affects health status, this book will consider the inputs, processes and outcomes of health services. Before you move on to study inputs, however, Chapter 2 will provide you with a brief introduction to the challenges that the planners and managers of health services face.

2 Challenges facing health services

Overview

The first part of this chapter will show that countries are increasingly concerned about the way health care is provided and that assessment and accountability have been the key drivers of recent health care reforms. The second part outlines the contributions of health services research to our understanding of health care and to improving the management of services.

Learning objectives

After working through this chapter, you will be better able to:

- **analyse the pressures underlying recent changes in health systems**
- **identify common goals of these reforms**
- **outline the contribution of health services research to the organization and management of health services.**

Key terms

Corporate rationalizers A contemporary approach to management in which the organization (corporation) attempts to dominate professional autonomy through the use of measurement and data.

Environmental turbulence The ever changing external pressures on an organization and its managers such as legislation, the national economy, professional associations and trades unions, and public opinion.

Gross national product (GNP) The market value of the goods and services produced by the nationals of a country irrespective of where they reside (i.e. includes expatriates and excludes resident foreigners).

Health services research (HSR) A multidisciplinary activity to improve the quality, organization and management of health services. HSR is not itself a discipline.

Payers (funders) The people who provide funds to pay for health care. In a tax-based system, the tax payers; in a social insurance system, employees and employers.

Professional autonomy The freedom that professionals have to make decisions without being accountable to their employers or the state.

Prospective payment Paying providers before any care is delivered, based on predefined activity levels and anticipated costs.

Providers Organizations (hospitals, health centres) or individuals (community nurses) who provide care.

Purchasers Those who purchase health services from providers on behalf of those eligible to use health care. In public systems this may be government or public bodies; in social insurance systems, the insurance company or sick fund.

Retrospective payment Paying providers for any work they have undertaken, with no agreement in advance.

The changing pattern of health care

Governments in most countries are concerned about the way health care is provided and reforms are high on the policy agenda. Why have pressures for reform built up over time? To understand the current problems of health services, you need to analyse the political and economic factors that are driving these changes. Arnold Relman, formerly editor of the *New England Journal of Medicine*, encapsulated the key concerns of health care policy in an article written at the end of the 1980s. Though based on US experience, he describes some of the universal problems of health services, and you may find parallels to your country.

 Activity 2.1

As you read the following edited version of the article by Relman (1988), identify the stages the author describes and take notes of factors that have contributed to growing expenditure. Don't worry about the economic terms: these will be explained later in the book.

When you have read the article you should be able to answer the following questions.

1 Describe the key features of each of Relman's eras of health care.
   • era of expansion
   • era of cost containment
   • era of assessment and accountability
2 How did the new funding arrangements, which were introduced in the 1960s, influence development of health services in the USA?
3 Why was cost control alone not considered as a successful strategy for managing health services and what criteria does the author suggest for evaluating health services?

 Assessment and accountability: the third revolution in medical care

Since the end of World War II the United States has seen two revolutions in its medical care system. It is now on the threshold of a third. The first of these began in the late 1940s and early 1950s and continued through the 1960s. It can be described as the era of expansion and was characterized by rapid growth in hospital facilities and the number of physicians, new developments in science and technology, and the extension of insurance coverage to the majority of the population. Medical schools increased and produced an army of new specialists trained in the use of sophisticated technology. The National Institutes of Health poured large resources into basic and clinical research, generating exciting advances that raised public interest and expectations. With the passage of Medicare and Medicaid legislation in 1966, nearly 85 percent of Americans had some form of medical insurance and the goal of universal access to health care seemed close at hand. A final and very important feature of this era was the appearance of investor-owned medical care businesses, mainly hospital chains, which were attracted by the opportunities for profit offered by the open-ended system of insurance payment and the expansion of medical services.

These developments led inevitably to the second revolution, which may be called the revolt of the payers or the era of cost containment. More specialists and more technology, many new hospital beds, and a rapidly growing system of health insurance plans that reimburse charges are an explosively inflationary mixture, so it was hardly surprising when per capita medical costs, even after correction for the cost of living, began to rise rapidly. Within two decades after Medicare began, the cost of care had risen from about 4 percent to more than 11 percent of the gross national product, and the trajectory of medical inflation still shows no signs of flattening. At first the third-party payers simply paid the bills, but then employers and the federal government revolted against the costs, and the new era of cost containment began. The result was prospective payment and managed care, as manifested by diagnosis-related groups and health maintenance organizations. Hospitals, formerly in a position to collect whatever they charged, suddenly found themselves facing tougher, monopolistic payers who now were dictating prices. Some states have instituted closely regulated global budgeting for hospitals, and some have established tight controls on new construction. The federal government has said that it prefers to depend on market competition rather than regulation, but market forces have limited application and dubious ethical standing in health care, and in any case, there is no evidence that competition has been any more successful in keeping costs down than other approaches ... The chief cause of the cost crisis is not so much the price as the ever increasing volume and intensity of medical services being provided in outpatient settings and hospitals.

Compounding the frustration of the third-party payers in their efforts to control costs is a growing worry about the unknown quality and outcomes of medical services. Furthermore, the discovery of large geographical variations in the incidence of certain services, unaccompanied by any discernible difference in outcome, has led to the suspicion that in many cases we still have much to learn about the indications for a given course of action or the reasons for choosing one procedure over another. It is bad enough, the payers say, to be confronted with uncontrollable medical costs, but the situation becomes intolerable if in addition no one knows what benefits accrue from the services we pay for or the quality of those services. To control costs, without arbitrarily reducing access to care or lowering the quality of care, we will have to know a lot more about the safety, appropriateness, and effectiveness of drugs, tests, and procedures and the way care is provided by our medical care institutions and professional personnel.

... Now, however, we appear to be entering a new era, as a strong new consensus on the need for assessment and accountability seems to be building. At an invitational conference

... a few months ago, representatives from government, private insurers, major corporations, community agencies, and the medical profession met to discuss the problem. There was remarkable unanimity on the conclusion that the time for a new national health care initiative had come. All agreed that to provide a basis for decisions on the future funding and organization of health care, we will have to know more about the variations in performance among institutions and medical practitioners and what these may mean. We will also need to know much more about the relative costs, safety, and effectiveness of all the things physicians do or employ in the diagnosis, treatment, and prevention of disease. Armed with these facts, physicians will be in a much stronger position to advise their patients and determine the use of medical resources, payers will be better able to decide what to pay for, and the public will have a better understanding of what is available and what they want.

This theme was sounded by Dr. Paul Ellwood in his 1988 Shattuck Lecture, published in the Journal a few months ago. Ellwood calls for a major national program of 'outcomes management' by which he means a system linking medical management decisions to new, systematic information about outcomes. He says, correctly I believe, that such a program 'will not automatically favor a decrease or increase in health care expenditures,' but it will certainly improve the quality and effectiveness of health care and provide a much firmer base for future economic decisions.

... To achieve these objectives will require much new financial support and unprecedented cooperation among physicians, government, private insurers, and employers. No one should underestimate the size or difficulty of the task. However, the logical necessity of this new initiative seems clear. We can no longer afford to provide health care without knowing more about its successes and failures. The era of assessment and accountability is dawning at last; it is the third and latest – but probably not the last – phase of our efforts to achieve an equitable health care system, of satisfactory quality, at a price we can afford.

 Feedback

Your answers should be similar to these.

1 Relman's three-stage model can be described as follows:

Era of expansion, 1940–1960s. Rapid growth in hospital facilities and doctors. New specialties and new technology raised public expectations. Policies removed the existing financial barriers to health care. New funding arrangements triggered the expansion of health services.

Era of cost containment, 1960s–1980s. The subsequent increase in demand led to a rapid growth of health care expenditure. Often spending grew faster than the national income and policy efforts were focused on cost control. Prospective payment systems started to replace retrospective payment as purchasers of health care began to challenge providers' supremacy.

Era of assessment and accountability, 1990s onwards. Ever-rising costs showed that cost control alone was not effective. Policies of the third era aim to improve the effectiveness and efficiency of service delivery and use by ensuring that care is appropriate (i.e. the benefits outweigh the costs).

2 With the introduction of Medicare and Medicaid in 1966, insurance coverage was extended to 85% of the US population, leading to a rapid growth in the number of people having access to health care. As reimbursement of care had barely any constraints, the number of new health service providers increased rapidly as well. Providers were attracted by the prospects of the open-ended system of insurance payments.

3 A focus on cost control alone could arbitrarily reduce access to care or lower the quality of services provided. For example, denying a new drug on grounds of higher cost alone might be unwise. Reasons to choose one treatment over the other should consider their relative cost-effectiveness. For example, while a new drug might be more expensive than an existing one it might be worth introducing if it is also more cost-effective. It could provide better value than a cheaper drug, for example by saving money in other areas of care. (Don't worry if this is unfamiliar to you. You will explore further the economic perspective in other books in the series.)

The essential point here is that health care should be:

- appropriate (effective and safe)
- humane (acceptability to patients)
- equitable (based on a person's need).

Relman argues that the third (and current) era (after expansion and cost containment) aims 'to achieve an equitable health care system, of satisfactory quality, at a price we can afford'.

What can health services research contribute to management?

In achieving the goal of an equitable health care system, of satisfactory quality, at a price we can afford, research and management play important roles. You need to distinguish between health services research (HSR) and investigations that managers perform in the planning and monitoring of health services. Both activities are important, but what is the difference?

1 Researchers aim to make findings that can be *generalized* – for example, in a study to find the optimum distance between health centres, researchers may aim to discover the right principles.
2 Investigations related to planning and management are of interest in a *particular* situation. An example would be an investigation into where exactly to site health centres in a particular country or an audit to assess the quality of care being provided in a particular hospital.

There is clearly an interactive relationship between management and HSR. As a manager, you would apply results from research and engage in management activities that may give rise to new research.

The scope and contribution of HSR has been outlined in an article by a British researcher, Nick Black (1997). While reading the following edited version, focus on the relationship between management and research and the potential of research to support management. The article introduces the concept of 'environmental turbulence', a useful framework for analysing and understanding the external pressures any manager will be under.

Health services research: saviour or chimera?

Crises in health services are rarely out of the news. But predictions of impending catastrophe are nothing new (for example, 18th century teaching hospitals felt they were doomed by the rising cost of leeches) and are not confined to countries with highly restricted publicly funded services. Do such crises result from incompetent management or merely indicate the magnitude of the task?

Although there will always be scope for improvements in management, the nature and scale of the task mean that troubles are inevitable. Managers face challenges from both within and outwith their organisations. The internal environment presents three major difficulties. First, health care is highly complex: there are dozens of occupational groups employed in the provision of health care, often competing with one another; complexity also arises because no two patients are identical, which restricts standardized processing; and for many patients, management of their care requires multiple activities to be coordinated. Second, all this complexity is ever changing. And third, unlike many other such organisations, some employees, especially doctors, not only exercise enormous influence on how resources are used, but also have considerable autonomy.

The many external pressures to which health services are subjected have been described as 'environmental turbulence'. Four principal sources of such turbulence can be identified: (1) government, through financial controls, guidance on health-care strategies, and level of social welfare provision; (2) local opinion, local politicians, and consumer organisations; (3) organisations representing health-care staff, through terms and conditions of service, and training requirements; and (4) the medical-industrial complex, through the promotion of new technologies in which they have commercial interests. All are legitimate stakeholders. It was into this cauldron that health services research (HSR) was introduced in the 1980s. Although research on health services has been undertaken for several decades, it is only in the past 10 years that it has received a huge boost in several industrial countries, including the USA, Canada, and the UK. Why has this happened?

Three influential groups have their reasons and expectations. All payers feel that HSR can help to solve the perennial difficulty of containing increasing costs. Clinicians, smarting from the criticisms of the therapeutic nihilists who had argued that health services had little effect, or even caused more harm than good, believe that research on health care can provide evidence to counter such attacks. The public, whose expectations have rapidly risen with the growth of consumerism, are the third group. These trends have heralded the era of assessment and accountability. But how realistic are these expectations of HSR? Will HSR prove to be a saviour, as many hope and anticipate, or just a chimera, a mere wild fancy or unrealisable dream?

The aim of HSR is to provide unbiased, scientific evidence to influence health services policy at all levels so as to improve the health of the public. It is not a scientific discipline but draws on and uses a wide range of methods from several disciplines, including sociology, statistics, economics, epidemiology, psychology, and history. It also requires input from and an understanding of biology, medicine, nursing, and other clinical areas. HSR challenges the dominant biomedical model in which disease occurs, leading to illness, which is then treated. Although this lies at the heart of the matter, HSR also considers all the other determinants of use of health care. As such, it usually adopts a population perspective, by contrast with the clinical view focusing on individual patients. HSR therefore seeks answers to such questions as: how much health care should we have? How should services be funded? Who should receive services? And how well are services being provided?

What has HSR ever done for us? To answer this question I have restricted myself to examples in surgery . . .

HSR has identified the value of non-medical aspects of care. My example comes from a much neglected aspect, that of hospital architecture. In a delightful study from the USA, the effect of the view from their hospital window was studied inpatients undergoing cholecystectomy. Some were nursed with a view of trees, others with a view of a brick wall. Those with the view of trees required less analgesia, had better psychological adjustment, and had a shorter stay in hospital.

HSR has improved our understanding of who uses services and why. Many factors, apart from the presence of disease, have proved influential, including gender, distance from facilities, patients' knowledge, and clinicians' judgment. Higher rates of appendicectomy in women than in men have long been recognized. Why should this be so? The initial medical response was that females were more likely to develop appendicitis, but no supportive evidence has been forthcoming. The more likely explanations are, first, appendicitis-like symptoms are more common in females, probably arising from ovarian dysfunction. Second, there is evidence in some cultures of young women using the operation to prove their independence. And third, there is widespread availability of surgical services – the gender difference is more pronounced the higher the overall operation rate in a population.

. . . Surgical rates can also be affected by people's knowledge about the procedure. In the early 1980s there was growing concern in many countries about the high rate of hysterectomies. This was true of Switzerland, where the health office in one canton decided to take action. Rather than try to persuade gynaecologists to be more circumspect in their use of the procedure, they mounted a public information campaign. Two months after the campaign began, the rate started declining, eventually falling by 26%. No change was recorded over this period in a control canton.

The final determinant of use of services I want to consider is clinicians' judgment. In the 1920s in New York City, 1000 11-year-olds had their throats examined. Sixty-one percent proved to have had their tonsils removed. Of the other 39%, the examining doctor thought about half needed tonsillectomy; the half with healthy tonsils were examined by another doctor, who thought that half of them required surgery. Again, the healthy children were re-examined by yet another doctor who declared that half of them needed the procedure. After four examinations, only 65 of 1000 children would have escaped with their tonsils intact.

Such variation in clinical opinion is not solely a thing of the past. In the 1980s physicians in the USA and UK were asked to consider several hundred clinical situations and to decide on the appropriateness of coronary surgery. There was a considerable difference: US physicians judged surgery appropriate in more situations than did British physicians (62% vs 41%).

. . . HSR has identified ways of improving the organisation and management of services. One subject that attracts more public and political attention than any other is waiting lists. Despite best endeavours, waiting lists are a permanent feature of health services. Among several reasons for such lists, one is our poor understanding of how waiting lists function. Traditionally, clinicians, managers and researchers have believed that waiting lists partly reflect a linear queue and partly a mortlake, in which certain common conditions are sidelined. Attempts to reduce waiting lists which have assumed one or both of these models have often failed. Qualitative study of how waiting lists were being managed revealed that neither model provided a satisfactory account of what was going on. Instead, a list seemed more like a store in which participants – patients, surgeons, clerks, managers – were actively creating, negotiating, and structuring the list. Solutions have to take this concept into account if they are to prove successful.

So is HSR a saviour or a chimera: will it rescue health care from the seemingly impossible dilemmas it faces or will it prove to be no more than an unrealisable dream, a mere wild fancy at the end of the 20th century? HSR has much to contribute, but will never have all the answers. Advocates of rational scientific solutions will therefore have to avoid unjustified claims and engendering unrealistic expectations. HSR can and should only ever be an influence on policy. We must recognise the legitimate role of other forces in shaping health services and seek ways of working with the other parties. In addition, we must not forget that HSR is but a player in a great experiment. We live in a period in which the corporate rationalisers, for whom HSR plays a key part, are challenging the tradition of professional autonomy. Many of us believe such a challenge will lead to a brighter future. But it is only a belief and we may be proved wrong. And we must remember that HSR is the flavour of the decade. But how long will the era of assessment and accountability last? This is but the third revolution in health services. A fourth may be waiting in the wings, so we must take full advantage of the current opportunities.

 Activity 2.2

As you have seen, there are internal and external sources of pressure on health services managers. This activity provides an opportunity to reflect on these pressures and the relevance of HSR in your country.

1 What are the three internal pressures identified?
2 For each of the four main sources of external pressures on management (government; local interests; organisations representing staff; medical-industrial complex suggest one example of each based on your experience in health services.

Feedback

1 Health care is highly complex, which limits the extent to which care can be standardized; this complexity is ever changing; and some employees (notably doctors) exercise enormous influence and have considerable autonomy.

2 You probably found many examples along the lines of those given below.

Government: almost everywhere governments want managers to meet financial or political targets, for example to cut public spending or to implement new policies for health services.

Local interests: local politicians often challenge the views of both managers and central government, as may the local media.

Organizations representing staff: trade unions fighting for better working conditions and terms of payment; professional organizations influencing training and staffing.

Medical-industrial complex: pharmaceutical companies and other suppliers often promote their products with aggressive marketing and may even resort to bribery.

Though equally important for low, middle and high income countries, most health services research has been conducted in high income countries. With the increasing concerns about health care finance, governments have become more interested in HSR and a number of low and middle income countries have started HSR programmes. In countries with academic traditions in public health, HSR is frequently associated with public health schools. But research has also emerged in medical schools and social sciences faculties. You may also find HSR attached to large public institutions like social insurance companies or health care provider organizations. A general concern is that the link between research and management is weak, and it may take a long time for results to disseminate into practice. You need to be aware that much of the success of HSR relies on cooperation with clinicians and managers yet, by it nature, HSR tends to challenge established medical knowledge. Successful health services researchers therefore need good political skills as well as strong research abilities.

Summary

Health care reforms are high on the policy agenda of many countries. Three eras have been suggested to explain how the pressures for reform have built up over time. After an initial era of expansion of health services, rising costs were followed by an era of cost containment. The limited scope of cost containment as a goal changed in the 1980s and 1990s to concern about how to assess health services and hold them accountable to the public and those paying for them. The chapter has also explored the relationship between management and HSR and shown how a multidisciplinary research approach can contribute to improvement in the quality and organization of health services.

References

Black NA (1997) Health services research: saviour or chimera? *Lancet* 349: 1834–6.

Relman AS (1988) Assessment and accountability. The third revolution in medical care. *New England Journal of Medicine* 319: 1220–2.

3 | Formal and lay care

Overview

Before embarking on an analysis of the different inputs to formal services, it is important to be aware of its scope and boundaries. In this chapter you will focus on the distinction between formal and lay (or informal) care. After reading a short explanation of the different types and levels of formal care, you will explore some of the key issues in the debate on lay care. You will learn what lay care is and why it is relevant for understanding health services. You will also look at the different attitudes of the formal sector towards lay care.

Learning objectives

After working through this chapter, you will be better able to:

- **outline levels and types of health care**
- **distinguish between formal and lay care**
- **recognize lay care as a major influence on formal care.**

Key terms

Formal care Care provided by trained, paid professionals usually in a formal setting.

Lay care Care provided by lay people who have received no formal training and are not paid. It includes self-care, care by relatives, friends and self-help groups.

Medicalization The tendency of doctors increasingly to define areas as being 'medical' and thus subject to their influence and control in the belief that this is helpful (also referred to as 'medical imperialism').

Primary care Formal care that is the first point of contact for people. It is usually general rather than specialized, and provided in the community.

Secondary care Specialized care that often can only be accessed by being referred by a primary care worker. It is usually provided in local hospitals.

Self-help groups Groups of unpaid, self-taught people that offer solutions to health problems in a lay setting, based on mutual support between persons experiencing similar conditions.

Tertiary care Highly specialized care that often can only be accessed by referral from secondary care. It is usually proved in national or regional hospitals.

Scope and levels of health care

When asked to consider the inputs to health care, you may think immediately of doctors, nurses and hospitals. But, as you are no doubt aware, the spectrum of care is much broader and there are different ways of categorizing the activities.

First, it may be difficult to define the *scope* of health services, as many other activities also affect health. Education, housing and employment policies may have a greater impact on health than those that you might identify as health care activities. So it is important to consider health care as an activity with a *primary intention* to improve people's health, as opposed to other activities which, while they may have an indirect effect on health, do not have this as their primary intent. You also need to consider the *spectrum* of services which range from health promotion and disease prevention, through curative care, rehabilitation and long term care, to palliative care and custodial care.

Second, you need to distinguish between *levels* of care:

Primary care Formal care that is the first point of contact for people. It is usually general rather than specialized, and provided in the community, for example by community nurses or general practitioners.

Secondary care Specialized care that often can only be accessed by being referred by a primary care worker. It is usually provided in local hospitals, for example orthopaedic surgery or psychiatry.

Tertiary care Highly specialized care that often can only be accessed by referral from secondary care. It is usually proved in national or regional hospitals, for example cardiac surgery or secure accommodation for mentally ill offenders.

 Activity 3.1

Like many definitions, they are not watertight and exceptions exist. Can you suggest some health care activities that do not fit with these definitions?

 Feedback

There are exceptions in all countries. For example, people can refer themselves to a hospital (secondary care) if they are injured and need the casualty department or emergency room. Also, specialized care is increasingly being provided in the community – for example, outreach clinics run by specialists in primary care centres.

 Activity 3.2

This activity gives you an opportunity to explore the range of services in the region where you live. The focus of the exercise is to make you aware of potential imbalances between care for mental and physical illness and imbalances between different levels of care.

Referring to the region where you live, find out the institutions providing care for road traffic accidents and those providing care for people who are mentally ill. If you do not know about service provision in your area, you may need to ask somebody involved in local services. Complete Table 3.1

You should consider the following types of services:

- Curative (primary, secondary and tertiary care
- rehabilitation
- long term care
- custody

Feedback

You may have found that some types of institution do not apply in all cases (for example, custody is only for mentally ill offenders), or do not exist in your country (for example, institutions for long term care may be rare or missing in areas where families care for chronically ill or disabled relatives). If you live in a low income country, you may have found that the country cannot provide the whole spectrum of care. Many countries face imbalances between types and levels of care. For example, there may be excessive curative care and a lack of preventive or rehabilitation services. The different types of care may be financed through different mechanisms, creating problems of cooperation and leading to barriers of access to care.

Care for the mentally ill is a matter of humanitarian concern in many countries. In high income countries services for these patients used to be provided in large institutions, separated from the communities. Closing these asylums and bringing services for the mentally ill to the community has been a reform issue in recent decades.

Formal and lay care

Thus far you have looked at the different types of formal care. However, as you will see, health care extends beyond the formal sector. You may ask why it is important to study the relationship between formal and lay care.

1 You need to be aware that 80% of all care is provided by lay people. Figure 3.1 illustrates the dimensions and limits of formal care.
2 Studying lay care will help you understand care-seeking behaviour, which is an important determinant of the use of formal services.
3 Incorporating the lay perspective is essential to community participation and a sense of ownership of local health services (an issue explored further in Chapter 11).

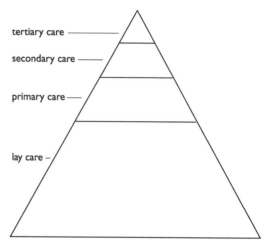

Figure 3.1 Formal and lay care

The roles of lay carers

Lay people may be involved in health care in three main ways:

- Providing information and advice as to what action someone might take. This might involve encouraging or discouraging someone to contact formal services. Lay referral cultures can have a significant impact on people's use of formal services.
- Emotional support. This might involve helping to buffer adverse life events which threaten someone's state of health, supporting changes in someone's behaviour that might affect their state of health (e.g. stopping smoking), or assisting and encouraging someone's recovery and rehabilitation after illness.
- Practical assistance in providing health and social care.

The last of these is the area of lay care that is closest to the services provided by formal carers. It also represents a 'grey area' where it can prove tricky to distinguish between the two sectors. There are three criteria that help distinguish lay from formal care:

1 The setting: formal care usually takes place in a formal setting (such as a health centre), while lay care usually takes place in an informal setting (such as a person's home).
2 The training: formal carers receive a formal training with some form of recognition at the end, whereas lay carers usually get no or only an unstructured training.
3 The rewards: formal carers are paid, whereas lay carers are usually not.

Activity 3.3

This activity is designed to help you reflect on the extent of lay care and who provides it.

1 Think of traditional healers or alternative therapists in your country. According to the above criteria, are they formal or lay carers?

2 Write down examples of lay care that exist in your country. Bear in mind that lay care covers a wide range of activities, including health promotion, nursing, diagnosis and treatment. What factors do you think determine the role of lay care in your country?

3 In your country, which members of the family would be most likely to care for an elderly disabled relative?

Feedback

1 You should have identified traditional healers or alternative therapists as formal carers. They have usually received some formal training and are usually paid.

2 You probably had no difficulty in finding a wide range of examples of lay care. You may have had some difficulty in deciding whether some particular candidates were lay or formal carers. The distinction can sometimes be difficult. Several factors determine the role of lay care: the level of economic development, views about the relative responsibilities of individuals and the state, cultural and religious beliefs, family structure (including geographical dispersion of families), and the power of the formal carers.

3 Lay care is provided mostly by women, and this appears to be a universal phenomenon.

The extent of lay care

Compared with formal care, little is known about lay care because few studies have been carried out and formal records are rarely kept. Despite this, it is clear that the majority of health care is provided by lay carers, in particular self-care and by family members. This is true regardless of a country's level of development.

In the UK, one-eighth of adults are carers to some extent. (This doesn't take into account routine parenting such as caring for a sick child.) While much of this activity is social care (washing, feeding, dressing), it also includes increasing numbers of people helping with the administration of formal health care by, for example, giving intravenous drugs (Kirk and Glendinning 1998; Pickard and Glendinning 2002). The contributions of men and of women were clear in a study of couples caring for a disabled relative. Women spent on average 3 hours each day, whereas their husbands contributed only 13 minutes. The same applies to care for children. In another study, of 400 couples both working full-time as doctors, 80% of the men viewed the wife as responsible for caring for their children when their child was sick.

Most people make use both of formal and lay care. We learn from an early age how to determine which is appropriate in different situations. Just think for a moment what you would do if you woke with abdominal pain. If it was mild you might decide to do nothing and see if the pain passed. If it persisted you might self-medicate with some medicine available 'over the counter' from a shop, or consult a friend or family member. If it still continued you might refer yourself to a formal carer such as a doctor. The decision as to which sector to use is not fixed but will vary with the condition. It will also depend on the services available, which in turn will be determined by the level of economic development as well as other factors.

The following article by Roland Msiska *et al.* (1997) describes the diversity of options for people living in Zambia who are suffering from a sexually transmitted disease (STD). The researchers were attempting to find out what determined people's choices.

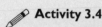

Activity 3.4

While reading, make notes on (1) the care options available and (2) the factors that influenced people's decisions to use either lay or formal care.

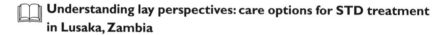

Understanding lay perspectives: care options for STD treatment in Lusaka, Zambia

Introduction

Studies conducted in the developing and developed world have identified several determinants for health care seeking behaviour patterns for various types of illness. These include type and severity of symptoms, the course of illness, sick role, perception regarding cause of illness, age, sex, education and economic status, social cost, social networking and lay referral mechanisms, availability of the service and their opinion of the efficacy of therapeutic options. These factors interact in a complex and diverse manner, and vary in their direction and power of influence on the behaviour of individuals or communities.

The objective of this study was to determine lay persons' perspectives in care seeking behaviour patterns for STD in selected sub-populations in Lusaka.

Methods

A combination of 20 unstructured interviews, 10 focus group discussions and four STD illness simulations were performed in purposively selected sub-populations with a varied age and sex mix in order to obtain information on health care seeking behaviour patterns.

. . . In general, the problem of HIV/AIDS was perceived as a greater and far more serious threat than other STDs, and little linkage was recognized between the two conditions. The commonest STDs identified were syphilis (*kaswende*), gonorrhoea ('leakage' or pus) and chancroid (*bola bola*), all of which were considered treatable with 'proper medicine'. Of interest is the fact that in spite of this knowledge, people believed that traditional medicine was still relevant in ensuring a satisfactory outcome in addition to hospital treatment. Traditional medicine is usually obtained from friends or older men and women who are conversant in the treatment of STDs.

Participants preferred private facilities to public health facilities – this includes private general practitioners, private chemists, street vendors and market stalls. Street and market vendors had an array of medicines which they prescribed according to the clients' description of the STD. The reasons for not wanting to use public health institutions for STD treatment were mainly the social costs and 'inconvenience' associated with hospitals and clinics rather than economic constraints (after all, as participants indicated, in Lusaka the GPs are far more expensive than the public health institutions). According to the clients, the set-up of the STD service at the University Teaching Hospital did not encourage them to go there because it was too cumbersome and left people vulnerable to exposure and embarrassment. For example, a client has to describe his/her symptoms to several health workers (including guards controlling the queues!) before reaching the right clinic. Derogatory remarks by staff, especially those attributing STD to lack of or loose morals, also contributed to the reluctance to attend the service. Compulsory partner attendance as a pre-condition to treatment also discouraged clients. In contrast to the public health institutions, GPs and street vendors tended to provide a quick 'no-questions-asked' service that appealed to and was approved by clients.

A total of four STD case simulations were carried out in private pharmacies. The results indicate that the sale of antibiotics for STDs has become a roaring and lucrative business in the compounds. Little or no information is provided to the buyer on the use of the drugs or on the type of drug being given. Of all the four pharmacies visited, only one refused to sell antibiotics without a doctor's prescription. The street vendors sold all kinds of antibiotics with little regard for packaging, duration or instructions for use. The amount of drug sold depended on the amount of money the client had.

Discussion

Patterns for STD care

Earlier studies in Lusaka revealed that options open to the sick 'are of bewildering complexity. They include . . . consultations with relatives, with white, Indian or fellow African employees of diverse tribal and linguistic origins; with neighbours and friends . . . Western doctors' (Frankenberg and Leeson 1976). The 10 focus group discussions and the 20 unstructured interviews in the bars confirm the diversity and complex nature of the care options, which in the case of STD include an array of options. These include self-medication, traditional healers, medicines sold in the markets and streets, as well as injections administered in the compounds. Private clinics, health centres and hospitals also provide a service, though the latter are perceived by clients to provide a less satisfactory service. As for drugs used in the treatment of STDs, these were widely available in the markets, stores and pharmacies. These antibiotics were being prescribed without any sort of regulatory framework and in circumstances that posed danger and doubt for the patient's successful treatment. This has the potential to cause drug resistance, thus further complicating the prevention of STD in Zambia.

Self-care

The term 'self-care' has diverse interpretations. The definition used in this study is that of Levin in which he describes self-care as 'a process by which people function on their own behalf in health promotion and prevention and in disease detection and treatment at the level of the primary resource in the health care system' (Levin 1981). This is further elaborated by John Fry into four elements of self-care, namely: health maintenance, self-medication, self-treatment, and participation in professional care. In all the 10 focus groups and 20 unstructured interviews, self-care was a predominant option in dealing with STDs. Self-care is particularly important in STDs due to the shame and stigma and social cost attached to the management of the illness.

Although there is little consistency in the definition of self-care among researchers, studies have shown that as much as 65–85% of health care is self-care. In the absence of studies on the quality of self-care that STD patients are providing for themselves, there is a potential danger of the emergence of resistant strains of STD organisms, of partially treated STDs and hence of increased complications. On the other hand, self-care pro-vides an opportunity for universal coverage for STD treatment in a resource-constrained environment such as Zambia. In the words of Levin, 'strengthening self-care . . . seems to represent a basic thrust towards a more adequate, more accessible, more dignified, and possibly more effective mode of using health resources, irrespective of the particular health delivery or financing system or, for that matter, political environment'. Strengthening self-care in Zambia provides an opportunity for the full partnership of lay persons and professionals in health care, consistent with the overall thrust of the health reform.

Factors influencing care seeking behaviour

The factors identified as influencing care seeking behaviour are: lay referral mechanisms, social cost, availability of option of care, economic factors, beliefs, stigma and quality of care as perceived by the users.

Lay referral mechanisms

As may be expected for an illness such as STD, exchange of information on STDs occurred within age and sex groups. Stigma and social cost associated with STDs made it difficult for students to consult elders on how to manage STDs once afflicted. Peer consultation was identified as the predominant approach among the students once infected with STDs.

Social cost

Social cost refers to 'the restructuring of personal relationships, customary exchange patterns and friendship ties that often accompany innovation'. The evidence from this study suggests that social cost is higher for female STD patients than male patients, in that although women preferred to be examined by female staff they were still being examined by men. The majority of clinical officers in Zambia are male and these are usually the front-line in the screening of STD patients.

Other aspects of social cost identified by all groups included being required to bring partners before STD treatment would be provided and the lack of privacy. The process of reducing social cost is reflected by the patients' preference for traditional healers rather than medical staff. The female participants observed that 'traditional healers would not request you to undress before providing you with treatment or insist that you need to bring a partner before giving one treatment'. Traditional healers rarely asked 'too many questions', as one participant said.

Expression of stigma

STD in the participating communities is highly stigmatized; it is associated with the use of labels such as *fimbusu* (literally translated as toilets) and *hule* (prostitutes). In all focus groups these terms were mainly used in relation to women suffering from STD, not men. Terms used to describe men suffering from STD had less offensive labelling, for example *kubukinsa*, which in literal translation means having an accident. In one focus group, females indicated that suffering from an STD was worse than having a child out of wedlock! This influences not only the recognition of symptoms but also the process of consultation and care seeking patterns.

Gender

As stated above, social cost is highest for female STD patients since the examining doctors tend to be male. Women were also disadvantaged by the requirement to bring partners as a condition of receiving treatment.

Staff attitudes and the location of STD clinics made it difficult for patients to access the health facilities within the area studied. Social culture expectations of women make this process particularly difficult for them.

Problems associated with use of government health centres and hospitals

In order to understand what is lacking in professional care from the groups' perspective, all groups were asked what they thought were the difficulties involved in obtaining treatment for STDs at government health centres and hospitals. The following emerged as problems: shortage of drugs, lack of privacy, long queues, being examined by a member of the opposite sex, high medical fees, demanding the attendance of the partner before provision of treatment. Focus group participants were unanimous in their opinion that the shortage of drugs was a creation of the health centre medical staff. This was confirmed, in their view, by the fact that some medical staff were 'selling' them drugs for STD treatment in the compounds.

 Feedback

1 You should have noted the following lay care options available: self-care, friends, older men and women. The formal care options were: private general practitioners, private chemists, street vendors and market stalls, public clinics and hospitals.

2 The factors that influenced people's choice included: lay referral mechanisms, social cost, availability of care options, economics, beliefs, stigma and the perceived quality of the care on offer.

Is the extent of lay care changing?

The connection between kinship obligation and caring is changing in most societies. One of the views held is that with the rise of modern industrial societies and integration of women into the labour market, family obligations are becoming weaker and are confined to the nuclear family. As a result, a larger number of elderly people live alone, and this increases the need for formal care. But it is important to be aware that throughout the world there is a willingness to care on the part of families and, indeed, most of the care for the elderly is provided by lay carers.

A second view is that there are fewer opportunities for lay care as families get smaller in size and greater geographical mobility separates family members. In addition, in some societies older people chose to live apart from their younger relatives, often alone if economic resources allow.

Formal carers' attitudes to lay care

There have been a variety of responses to the emergence over the last few decades of a more vociferous and confident lay sector. Three types of attitude can be discerned:

1 There is a range of activities that should only be performed by formal carers with adequate knowledge and training. Formal care therefore needs to expand and take over lay care. This view may be associated with a fear that a vibrant lay sector could be used to cut spending on formal care. The extension of medical involvement in people's lives is referred to as *medicalization*.
2 Lay carers are capable of being trained by formal carers to carry out specific tasks that formal carers determine. In other words, the extent of lay care is determined and 'granted' by formal carers.
3 Lay carers should be encouraged and supported by formal carers. Given the overwhelming needs for care in the population, a small formal sector cannot cope without an alliance with lay carers. Unlike the preceding attitude, the independence of lay carers is encouraged rather than restricted and controlled. Lay contributions are seen as an opportunity rather than a threat.

Summary

Health care encompasses a wide range of activities with a primary intention to improve health. The distinction between formal and lay care is important for understanding the scope of health care. The major part of care is provided by the lay sector in an informal setting and is unpaid. Lay care is a major determinant of the amount of formal care consumed. It can take a range of different forms: individual self-care; care within families and social networks; and self-help groups. You have explored key issues in the changing relation between kinship obligation and care and attitudes of the formal sector towards lay care.

References

Frankenberg R, Leeson J (1976) Disease, illness and sickness: social aspects of the choice of healer in a Lusaka urban community, in London JB (ed.) *Social Anthropology and Medicine*. New York: Academic Press.

Kirk S, Glendinning C (1998) Trends in community care and patient participation: implications for the roles of informal carers and community nurses in the United Kingdom. *Journal of Advanced Nursing* 28: 370–81.

Levin LS (1981) Self-care in health: potentials and pitfalls. *World Health Forum* 2: 177–84.

Msiska R, Nangawe E, Mulenga D, Sichone M, Kamanga J, Kwapa P (1997) Understanding lay perspectives: care options for STD treatment in Lusaka, Zambia. *Health Policy & Planning* 12: 248–52.

Pickard S, Glendinning C (2002) Comparing and contrasting the role of family carers and nurses in the domestic health care of frail older people. *Health & Social Care in the Community* 10: 144–50.

SECTION 2

Inputs to health care

4 Diseases and medical knowledge

Overview

You have seen why this book takes a systems approach to the analysis of health services, read about the pressures underlying current health services and examined the role of health services research in the process of change. This chapter and the next three cover the various inputs to formal health care.

In the previous chapter you saw that lay care has a major influence on formal care. You will now explore the concepts of diseases and medical knowledge, which are fundamental to understanding health services. You will learn what disease is and how categories of diseases change over time. You will also explore how cultural factors affect medical knowledge and how this contributes to our understanding of international differences between health services.

Learning objectives

By the end of this chapter you will be better able to:

- **outline the concept of 'disease' and describe how it relates to social and cultural factors**
- **describe the generation of medical knowledge and give examples of how categories of diseases arise**
- **analyse the relationship between culture and medicine and exemplify how cultural factors affect international comparison.**

Key terms

Culture The values, beliefs and attitudes associated with a social system.

Disease A condition which, judged by the prevailing culture, is painful or disabling and deviates from either the statistical norm or from some idealized status.

Diseases Patterns of factors (symptoms, signs) that occur in many people in more or less the same way.

Felt need A person's subjective assessment of their need for better health.

Normative need A professional assessment of a person's need for health care based on objective measures.

Pathological Relating to form or function that is deemed to be abnormal.

Physiological Relating to bodily function (such as breathing) that is deemed to be 'normal'.

Introduction

Health services are often described and studied in terms of disease groups or patients' groups as though these categories were unproblematic. This is not so. It is necessary to consider two questions:

- What is disease?
- What are diseases?

What is disease?

You may think that the answer to this is straightforward: disease is what doctors define to be ill health. But the concept of 'disease' is more complex and is fundamental to understanding health services.

You could define 'disease' as the absence of health and health as the absence of disease. But this is circular. Defining 'disease' involves two approaches, self-assessment and professional assessment. *Self-assessment* inevitably involves a subjective assessment of how one feels about one's own health. Therefore, it is often referred to as 'felt need' and is an indication of a person's 'need for health'. Given that such an assessment is subjective, we will vary in our perceptions. At one extreme there are stoics who will put up with more than others. In contrast, there are people who are hypochondriacal and will complain about the slightest problem. Also, lay people may not distinguish between symptoms of disease and symptoms that are normal or physiological such as those associated with pregnancy or teething.

Professional or *biomedical assessment* is based on objective, scientific and often statistically based definitions of illness. Biomedical observation uses signs and test results to define disease. Professional definitions also encompass whether or not a cost-effective treatment exists. In other words, it is a definition of a person's 'need for health care'. It is sometimes referred to as 'normative need'. Despite the sophisticated methods used, it can still be difficult for professionals to say that disease is either present or absent as most measures are *continuous* (such as a blood sugar level) rather than *dichotomous* (whether a bone is fractured or not) variables.

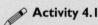 **Activity 4.1**

In 1954 Lester King, an American doctor, explored the distinction between subjective and objective definitions of disease. As you will see, King defines disease as 'the aggregate state of those conditions which, judged by the prevailing culture, are deemed painful or disabling, and which, at the same time, deviate from either the statistical norm or from some idealized status'. As you read the following extract from his article, write down an example for each of the following statements:

1 Disease varies with cultural context.
2 There are painful conditions which are not considered as disease.
3 There is deviance from a statistical norm which is not deemed pathological.
4 A deviance from an idealized state could be a disease although it doesn't deviate from the statistical norm.

What is disease?

As illustrating the confusion surrounding the notion of disease, I recall a very precise young physician who asked me what our laboratory considered the normal hemoglobin level of the blood (with the particular technique we used). When I answered, '12 to 16 grams, more or less,' he was very puzzled. Most laboratories, he pointed out, called 15 grams normal, or perhaps 14.5. He wanted to know how, if my norm was so broad and vague, he could possibly tell whether a patient suffered from anemia, or how much anemia. I agreed that he had quite a problem on his hands, and that it is a very difficult thing to tell. So difficult, in fact, that trying to be too precise is actually misleading, inaccurate, stultifying to thought, and philosophically very unsound.

He wanted to know why I didn't take one hundred or so normal individuals, determine their hemoglobin by our method, and use the resulting figure as the normal value for our method. This, I agreed, was a splendid idea. But how were we to pick out the normals? The obvious answer is, just take one or two hundred healthy people, free of disease . . . But that is exactly the difficulty. We think of health as freedom from disease, and disease as an aberration from health. This is travelling in circles, getting us nowhere.

. . . One way of determining health is by this subjective report. The man who says, 'I feel just fine,' may consider himself entirely sound. Conversely, he who complains of feeling 'terrible' may think of himself as seriously ill. These subjective impressions are essential, and highly significant, but they are not entirely reliable. Here we come up against the distinction between what 'seems' and what 'really is,' between 'appearance' and 'reality.' We are all familiar with the man who had periodic routine examinations, who passed all tests, who felt subjectively fine, and who suddenly dropped dead. Or the man with no complaints at all but, cajoled into a routine chest X-ray, found he has a symptomless cancer. In such cases the individual 'seemed' healthy, subjectively he felt healthy, but 'really' he wasn't.

To understand health or disease we must have some objective measurements in addition to the introspective account. If we can weigh or measure something, then we have a little more confidence, and we feel more firmly grounded in objective reality. And there is no end of different features that we can thus quantitate. With the help of measurements and statistical analysis we can get a very whole picture of what exists and in what distribution, and, moreover, what we may reasonably expect in the future. But ordinarily statistics alone cannot label any part of the data as 'diseased.' When we apply statistical methods we already have in mind the idea of health. We exert selection on the cases we study. Thus, to find the 'normal' blood sugar level we eliminate known diabetics. And the basal metabolic rate, in health, we determine after omitting known thyroid disease.

In spite of the circularity, the concepts of health and disease belong together. There are

certain factors which are important for defining and distinguishing them. One is the subjective report, which is of only moderate reliability. The sense of well-being frequently
correlates with what we mean by health, but the correlation is not high, Certainly a sense
of well-being does not preclude the prevalence of disease, while the absence of such
subjective feeling does not indicate disease.

Another important factor is the statistical distribution, quite independent of any subjective
report. Let us imagine, for example, a statistical study of body temperature, on completely
random samples. We would find an overwhelming majority of individuals within a narrow
band, between 98 and 99°F. However, a very small percentage will show much higher
figures, such as 102°, 101°, or 105°, or more. These individuals who depart from the norm,
are by definition abnormal. This deviation, by itself, does not make them diseased. Thus,
persons with an intelligence quotient of 180, or with the ability to run 100 yards in 9.4
seconds, are also highly abnormal. However, when a deviation is tied up with malaise, pain,
or death, or is intimately associated with conditions which lead to disability or death, then
the abnormality forms part of disease.

Statistical norms, even when correlated with malaise, can furnish only a part of the total
picture. For example, statistics can establish the normal body temperature and, by correlation with malaise, pain, or death, the desirable body temperature. But in the matter of, say,
dentition, the statistical norm does not define the healthy or the desirable. Very few native
Americans possess thirty-two intact, well-aligned teeth. Yet when we speak of sound or
healthy dentition we have in mind the ideal of thirty-two intact, well-aligned teeth. In this
case it is deviation from the *ideal* which constitutes disease, not deviation from a statistical
norm.

These ideals stem from two sources. One is concrete observation. Nothing can serve as a
model of health unless it has been an observed characteristic or feature. And second, any
such feature must be an object of general desire, possessing value which appeals to the
mass of the population. One person might desire to be eight feet tall, yet the majority of
people do not. The ideals of height, of weight, of bust measurement, or head size, that is, the
range which the majority desires, vary from one nation or tribe to another, and from one
generation to another. Changes in diet, for example, can in a few generations change the
ideals in regard to stature. But at the present time a height of eight feet is not a matter of
general craving.

. . . Disease lies in the realm of pain, discomfort, or death. There are, however, many
examples of pain and discomfort which we cannot so designate. A teething infant or a
woman in childbirth is suffering pain. We may try to relieve this pain, but we do not think of
teething or childbirth as diseases. We call them normal functions. To be a healthy infant is
to go through a period of teething. We conclude that discomfort which constantly attends
a normal desirable function and is intimately or essentially bound up with that desirable
function is not in the realm of disease.

It follows that our concepts of disease are very closely related to our values. Frequently
our values may be severely determined by convention. China, for example, did not regard
as diseased those upper-class women whose feet were bound, and who thereby suffered
pain and diminution in function. Our contemporary culture takes a different view which
means that our conventions and values of health are different from the Chinese. In most of
our western civilization the seeing of visions we consider a sign of a diseased state. But in
some epochs of our civilization the seer of visions was a leader in the community, receiving
special honor because of his unusual endowment. Certainly the egregious and unusual, the

literally abnormal, represent disease only if judged by indigenous cultural values. Convention plays a very important part in shaping our values. And the quantity of our knowledge plays a very important part in shaping our conventions.

Disease is the aggregate of those conditions which, judged by the prevailing culture, are deemed painful or disabling, and which, at the same time, deviate from either the statistical norm or from some idealized status. Health, the opposite, is the state of well-being conforming to the ideals of the prevailing culture, or to the statistical norm. The ideal itself is derived in part from the statistical norm, and in part from the abnormal which seems particularly desirable.

 Feedback

1 You may have thought of foot binding in traditional Chinese society or low blood pressure, considered a disease in Germany but not elsewhere.

2 Teething, childbirth.

3 Obviously a number of biomedical parameters vary without being related to pathology – for example, a high blood sugar level after a meal does not imply diabetes.

4 Dental health in a population of elderly people – though the number of teeth lost does not deviate from the statistical norm (as all in that age group have fewer teeth), the condition deviates from the idealized state.

Other examples of how the boundary between being healthy and being diseased vary between places and over time are:

* malaria – in Europe any person with a parasitaemia (presence of malaria parasites in the blood) would be treated, whereas in tropical endemic areas where 60% of the population may have a parasitaemia but no symptoms, only persons with manifest disease would be treated;
* dyslexia, chronic fatigue syndrome and repetitive strain injury – have all been recognized as diseased states in recent years whereas previously they were not;
* homosexuality – used to be categorized by the World Health Organization as a diseased state.

What are diseases?

Having explored the concept of disease, you will now look at the different ways of categorizing diseases. Why is this important? Imagine you want to assess how the health care costs for patients with coronary heart disease have changed during recent decades. You might analyse medical records by looking at diagnoses. But which diagnoses should you choose? Ischaemic heart disease, degenerative heart disease, angina pectoris, myocardial infarction, coronary sclerosis and coronary insufficiency are all terms you may find in the records. Your results will depend on the definition you adopt.

Medical knowledge is based on categorizing states of ill health into discrete diseases. Diseases are patterns of factors (symptoms, signs) that occur in many people in more or less the same way. But where do the particular categories that we use

come from? One way of understanding a complicated system such as disease categorization is to study it when changes occur. Changes occur for five reasons:

1 Real changes in occurrence – for example, newly emergent diseases such as HIV/
   AIDS and new variant Creutzfeldt–Jacob disease. Diseases may also disappear –
   for example, sweating sickness (English sweat), which occurred in five epidemics
   between 1486 and 1551 and then disappeared; endemic Tyrolean infantile cir-
   rhosis, which lasted from 1900 to 1974; and encephalitis lethargica, which
   appeared in Europe and North America between 1919 and 1926. (Of interest and
   considerable concern is the fear that the latter may be reappearing in the
   twenty-first century.)

2 Changes in name – many different names were used for the same disease before
   the name coronary heart disease had been created, as mentioned above
   (Stehbens 1987). Glue ear (otitis media with effusion) is another example: the
   name for the same condition has changed more than 50 times since the
   nineteenth century (Black 1984).

3 Changes from single to multiple categories – this is a common phenomenon
   with the progress of medical knowledge. For example, diabetes was first split
   into diabetes insipidus and diabetes mellitus on the basis of the appearance and
   taste of the patient's urine. The latter was then divided into type I and type II on
   whether or not the problem was the failure of the person to create insulin or the
   failure of their body to respond to insulin. More recently, molecular biology has
   contributed to further subcategorization of diabetes.

   Another example is childhood diarrhoea in rural Bangladesh. While western
   medicine has no subdivisions, four types are well recognized by local people:
   ajirno (caused by indigestion and food poisoning, accounting for about 50% of
   cases); *arnasha* (contains mucus, cause unknown, and accounting for 33% of
   cases); *dud haga* (caused by ingesting contaminated breast milk, accounting for
   12% of cases); and a severe, watery dehydrating form accounting for 5% of cases
   (Chowdhury *et al.* 1988).

4 Changes in recognition of abnormality – this includes a range of conditions
   where medicine has changed its view. Examples include ptosis in the nineteenth
   century (the erroneous belief that the large bowel should not be free to move
   within the abdomen, leading to surgeons attaching the bowel to the abdominal
   wall) and night starvation in the 1930s (the belief that people suffered from low
   sugar levels as they slept and should, therefore, have a sugary drink before going
   to bed).

5 Uncovering of previously rare conditions – due to the reduction or elimination
   of other prevalent conditions. This is explained in the following extract from an
   editorial in the *Lancet* (1993):

   > The apparent newness of diseases has fuelled fierce debates. Many major
   > scourges of our 20th century industrialized world received their proper
   > names only in the second half of the last century or early in this one;
   > examples include coronary heart disease, schizophrenia, and rheumatoid
   > arthritis. Many doctors cannot credit that diseases which to us stand so
   > clearly on their own might have escaped the recognition of medical profes-
   > sionals of bygone times – hence the idea that these are diseases 'caused' by
   > civilisation. Medawar proposed an alternative view – that most diseases that
   > afflict us from middle age onwards might simply represent 'unfavourable'
   > genes that have accumulated to express themselves in the second half of our

lives. This could never be corrected by any evolutionary pressure since such pressures act only on the first half of our lives: once we have reproduced it does not greatly matter that we grow 'sans teeth, sans eyes, sans taste, sans everything'. Sexual attraction and physical vigour have served their turn and thereafter all types of haphazardly accumulated decay can freely express themselves. Civilisation, which has wiped out famine and pestilence in industrialized society, is therefore not the *cause* of our chronic diseases; it merely unveiled what our genes had lurking in store for us for centuries, if not millennia, as we now live long enough to see these genes massively expressing themselves. Such large-scale expression has greatly facilitated the 'discovery' of the diseases of civilisation – i.e., their description as separate entities. This notion finds support in the writings of historical demographers and historians who believe that our 'western' chronic disease pattern already existed among the few well-to-do people of the past, who were slightly better nourished, slightly more exempt from pestilences, and lived somewhat longer. If true, lifestyle changes will be of little avail.

While it is easy to point out examples of mistaken observations and beliefs in the past, we need to be cautious in our confidence about present-day knowledge. Scientific knowledge represents our best explanation and understanding of the world (both natural and social) at present – at best, scientific 'truth' is only historically relative and is conditional, that is, it will change in the future.

Culture and disease

As you have seen, the perception of disease has a cultural dimension, affecting both self-assessment and professional judgement. There is a large body of literature from medical anthropology describing the cultural context of disease. Many of the underlying differences in health services are due to cultural reasons.

What is culture?

Culture is a set values, beliefs and attitudes which are associated with a social system. For example, when comparing traditional Indian (Ayurvedic) medicine to western medicine, you may analyse the *material culture* and compare the medical tools and products used by both systems. You can also analyse the *non-material culture* and examine the ideas underlying Ajurvedic and western medicine. These ideas are the different *beliefs, values* and *norms*, which are reflected in medical theory and practice of both systems. You may, for example, compare the methods of generating medical knowledge and classifying diseases. Or you may compare the beliefs and norms underlying self-perception of disease in both cultures.

Activity 4.2

In her book, *Medicine and Culture*, published in 1988, Lynn Payer explored these differences from the perspective of a medical journalist who has studied health care in the

USA and Europe. As you read the following extract from her book, consider these questions:

1 What examples of international differences in treatment are cited?
2 What examples of international differences in diagnosis does Payer cite?
3 What implications do these differences have for health services research and management?

 Medicine and culture

My original interest in the subject of medical differences had been purely an intellectual one. But shortly after I had begun my research, a routine gynecologic checkup in France revealed a grapefruit-sized fibroid tumor in my uterus, a very common condition of women. While I rejected the suggestion of a colleague to become a sort of 'traveling tumor,' visiting doctors in a number of different countries to see what their treatment recommendations were, a recurrence of the fibroids after their initial removal by myomectomy after I had moved back to America gave me a chance to compare those two countries. In France, where great value is put on the woman's ability to bear children, hysterectomy was not even suggested as an option. Instead, the French surgeon told me I must have myomectomy, a major operation in which the fibroid tumor is removed while the ability to have children is preserved. I was told that six such operations could be performed without even necessitating a Cesarean section were I to become pregnant. In the United States I was put under a great deal of pressure for hysterectomy and told that a second myomectomy would be impossible. In neither case did the doctors seem to realize that their therapeutic recommendations were influenced less by the facts of my case than by how much the culture in which they operated valued the ability to have children.

World travelers who have had to see a doctor in a foreign country have usually discovered that medicine is not quite the international science that the medical profession would like us to believe. Not only do ways of delivering medical care differ from country to country; so does the medicine that is delivered. The differences are so great that one country's treatment of choice may be considered malpractice across the border.

Some of the most commonly prescribed drugs in France, drugs to dilate the cerebral blood vessels, are considered ineffective in England and America; an obligatory immunization against tuberculosis in France, BCG, is almost impossible to obtain in the United States. German doctors prescribe from six to seven times the amount of digitalis-like [heart] drugs as their colleagues in France and England, but they prescribe fewer antibiotics, with some German doctors maintaining antibiotics shouldn't be used unless the patient is sick enough to be in the hospital. Doses of the same drug may vary drastically, with some nationalities getting ten to twenty times what other nationals get. French people have seven times the chance of getting drugs in suppository form as do Americans. In the late 1960s American surgery rates were twice those of England; and the intervening years have seen this surgery gap widen, not close. Rates for individual operations vary even more. One study found three times as many mastectomies in New England as in England, even though the rate of breast cancer was similar; another found that German-speaking countries had three times the rate of appendectomies of other countries; there are six times the number of coronary bypasses per capita in America when compared to England. . . .

The same clinical signs may even receive different diagnoses. Often, all one must do to acquire a disease is to enter a country where that disease is recognized – leaving the country will either cure the malady or turn it into something else. The American schizophrenic of a few years ago might well have found his disease called manic-depressive disease or even neurosis had he sought a second opinion in Britain; in France he likely would have been diagnosed as having a delusional psychosis. The Frenchman suffering from spasmophilia or the German from vasovegetative dystonia would be considered merely neurotic in Britain or perhaps a victim of panic disorder in the United States if he were considered sick at all.

. . . One World Health Organization study found that doctors from different countries diagnosed different causes of death even when shown identical information from the same death certificates. There was a considerable amount of disagreement in coding infective and parasitic disease, 'other heart' diseases, hypertension, pneumonia, nephritis and nephrosis, and diseases of the newborn. 'There was fairly good agreement . . . on whether a death was due to a malignant neoplasm [cancer] or not, but less agreement on the location of neoplasms,' a finding confirmed by another study sponsored by the American National Cancer Institute.

. . . The widespread ignorance that medicine in highly developed countries can be so different has a number of serious implications. First, all sorts of unjustified conclusions are currently being drawn from international statistics. A press handout concerning rates of coronary artery disease in various countries, for example, showed the rate to be low in West Germany. While the person who compiled the release had copied the figures correctly from international statistics, he was unaware that while West Germany reports relatively low rates of coronary artery disease, the country reports much higher rates of 'other' heart disease than do England and the United States. If the rates of coronary artery disease and other heart disease are taken together, as it has been suggested they should, West Germany, England, and the United States have similar rates of heart disease.

Second, the different ways that different countries treat the same disease constitute a sort of natural experiment; yet because most people are unaware of the experiment in the first place, they are unable to draw the conclusions that might result. For example, French doctors have widely prescribed calcium for a number of years, and a closer examination of osteoporosis rates there might help illuminate the role of calcium in this disease . . .

Finally, many of the medical mistakes made in each country can be best understood by cultural biases that blind both the medical profession and patients, causing them to accept some treatments too quickly and other treatments reluctantly or not at all. Understanding the cultural basis for these mistakes can perhaps prevent them – or at least lessen their impact.

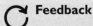 **Feedback**

1 International differences in treatment:

    a) Fibroids require hysterectomy in the USA but myomectomy in France.
    b) Cerebral vasodilators used in France but not in the UK and USA.
    c) BCG vaccination used universally in France but not in the USA.
    d) Higher use of heart drugs in Germany than in the USA, France and UK.
    e) Fewer antibiotics used in Germany than in France, the USA and UK.

f)   Suppositories used commonly in France but not in the USA, UK or Germany.

g)   Surgical rates vary between countries.

2 International differences in diagnosis:

a)   Schizophrenia (USA); manic depression or neurosis (UK); delusional psychosis (France).

b)   Neurosis (UK); spasmophilia (France); vasovegetative dystonia (Germany); panic disorder (USA).

3 Implications for HSR and management:

a)   Care required when making international comparisons of patterns of disease and use of health services.

b)   International variations can be used to compare the effectiveness and efficiency of different services.

c)   Understanding the cultural biases that may lead to fewer medical mistakes.

 Activity 4.3

Compare the drug consumption for different categories of diseases between the UK and Germany as shown in Table 4.1. Does it reflect the cultural differences between the two countries mentioned by Payer? Make brief notes on your comparison.

Table 4.1 Pharmaceutical consumption in the UK and Germany in defined daily doses in 1990

Indication	Germany	UK
Cardiovascular system	607	234
Respiratory system	583	435
Digestive system	511	406
Central nervous system	323	441
Systematic hormone replacement	28	59

Source: Fink-Anthe (1992)

Feedback

Though there are several important factors determining prescribing behaviour, such as guidelines, incentives and marketing efforts of the drug industry, some differences can only be explained by cultural reasons. The largest differences above relate to treatment of diseases of the cardiovascular and the central nervous system. The observed high level of cardiovascular drugs in Germany is consistent with Payer's view. The high levels of tranquillizers and antidepressants prescribed in the UK have been attributed to the cultural attitude of 'keeping a stiff upper lip' in personal troubles.

Summary

The concept of disease is dependent on social and cultural factors. Medical knowledge is based on categorizing states of ill health into discrete diseases. Analysing why these categories change over time provides insight into how medical knowledge is generated. In this chapter you have also learned about the cultural beliefs, values and norms underlying medical thinking. Cultural factors account for many of the differences observed in international comparison of health services.

References

Black NA (1984) Is glue ear a modern phenomenon? A historical review of the medical literature. *Clinical Otolaryngology* 9: 155–63.

Chowdhury M, Vaughan PV, Abed FH (1988) Use and safety of home-made oral rehydration solutions: an epidemiological evaluation from Bangladesh. *International Journal of Epidemiology* 17: 655–65.

Fink-Anthe C (1992) Kulturell beeinflußte Therapiegewohnheiten: Bedeutung für den europäischen Markt. *Deutsche Apotheker Zeitung* 29: 1534–9.

King L (1954) What is disease? *Philosophy of Science* 1: 193–203.

Lancet (1993) Rise and fall of diseases. *Lancet* 341: 151–2.

Payer L (1988) *Medicine and Culture*. New York: Henry Holt and Co.

Stehbens WE (1987) An appraisal of the epidemic rise of coronary heart disease and its decline. *Lancet* 1: 606–11.

5 Medical paradigms

Overview

In the previous chapter you saw how medical knowledge is generated. You learned that it is important to recognize that the notion of 'disease' is based on both subjective and objective assessment, and that these are influenced by the social and cultural environment. This chapter will extend the view to other aspects of medicine. You will explore the concept of medical paradigms, which will show how the concepts of illness have changed over time. This will help you to understand the roles of health care professionals and patients and some of the current critique of health services. You will also look more closely at the role of clinicians in the development of medical knowledge.

Learning objectives

After working through this chapter, you will be better able to:

- outline the concept of medical paradigms
- distinguish the major shifts in medical paradigms that have occurred in western medicine
- discuss the contributions that clinicians make to the development of medical knowledge and the limitations of these.

Key terms

Case series Study of a series of cases to identify common or recurring features.

Case study Observation and analysis of a single case to generate a hypothesis.

Discourse The way language is used in a particular area of social life.

Holism The conceptualization of a system as a whole and the belief that the whole is greater than the sum of the parts.

Medical cosmology The study of medical paradigms.

Medical paradigm The prevailing thoughts and knowledge about health and disease.

Reductionism Consideration of the component parts rather than the whole organism or organization.

Medical paradigms

As you have seen in the previous chapter, categories of diseases may change. Disease classification is just one aspect of medical knowledge. But, as you are probably aware, there are others, such as:

- aetiology (the cause of disease)
- pathogenesis (the way disease develops)
- pathology (the underlying fault or abnormality in a tissue or organ)
- natural history of disease (the way a disease develops and progresses)
- treatment.

At any given time, the prevailing thoughts and knowledge (the medical paradigm) need to be internally consistent if medical knowledge is to represent a set of coherent views on all aspects of medicine. These views relate not only to the conceptualization of illness but also to the research methods used, teaching approaches and, most important, the way health care practitioners perceive their patients. Conversely, these views also influence what patients expect from practitioners – they affect the patient-practitioner relationship. Importantly, too, medical views change over time, and at any one time they are just a manifestation of prevailing thoughts and knowledge. The totality of views at a given time constitutes the medical paradigm, the study of which has been referred to as 'medical cosmology'.

The importance of language

You need to be aware that the views held on a subject are related to the use of language. Indeed, one field of research focuses on examining written and spoken material to find out the underlying thought on a subject. For example, whether people have regarded madness as something evil, as divinely inspired or as mental illness has varied during history with the changing discourse on madness (as you will see in the example below).

The French philosopher Michel Foucault (1926–84) emphasized the importance of language for structuring knowledge and exerting power. To him, the way language (writing, talking) is used directs people to understand issues in certain ways that constitute their perception and knowledge of the world. He examined the development of language in certain areas of social life and how this process was used to exert power. He called the way language is used in a particular area *discourse*. Powerful groups can influence discourses in a particular area and, conversely, a particular discourse creates power by limiting the meaning of language.

In one of his key books, *Madness and Civilization* (1981), he explored the use of language, like an archaeologist digging through layer after layer and tracing how, in the western world, madness – which was once thought to be divinely inspired – came to be thought of as mental illness. He showed that, depending on the historical period, the mentally ill were treated as outcasts, and later were imprisoned and treated as criminals, before reforms in the nineteenth century led to humanitarian treatment in asylums and the rise of psychiatry as a profession.

Since then the discourse on madness has been dominated by psychiatry. But is it changing again? With the advent of effective drugs, much mental illness can be treated in the community. With decarceration from the large asylums that were a feature of nineteenth and early twentieth century care, professions other than psychiatry are gaining influence on the discourse, and the way in which people with these conditions are viewed has been gradually changing from 'inmates' to 'patients' and thence to 'clients'.

Why study changing discourse and shifts in the medical paradigm?

Why should you study the changing discourse on medicine and shifts in the medical paradigm? There are three reasons:

1 It helps you to understand the views held on patients and diseases.
2 It provides insight into some of the universal problems of modern health care, in particular the interaction between practitioners and patients.
3 As you will see later in this chapter, it helps you understand the strengths and limitations of clinical research.

Three major shifts in medical paradigms have occurred in western medical knowledge (Jewson 1976).

Bedside medicine

Before 1800, doctors' knowledge and their observation of patients were largely confined to visiting their middle and upper class patients in their own homes. The prevailing explanation of death and disease was imbalances in the four humours (key fluids) of the body – blood, choler (yellow bile), phlegm and black bile. This was a holistic view in which illness arose from a psychosomatic disturbance of the whole person. Doctors' understanding was based on speculation and inference, and their role was to predict the future (prognosis) and apply therapy, such as bleeding the patient.

Hospital medicine

In the nineteenth century, Europe and North America witnessed progressive urbanization of the population as people left the land and moved to the new, rapidly expanding cities which offered jobs and higher income. One consequence was the development of institutions to accommodate or simply contain the more unfortunate members of society who could not benefit from the new opportunities – the disabled, the elderly and the sick. A variety of measures were taken by local and national governments. From the point of view of medical knowledge, the gathering of large numbers of the sick poor in institutions plus the employment of doctors to provide rudimentary care gave the opportunity for groups of patients to be studied. The sick came under the 'clinical gaze', so that doctors could start to count things and observe associations and trends. In addition, when patients died, doctors could carry out post-mortems (autopsies) to see what had been going on (pathology). In addition, the physical sciences were making great advances and the application of new understanding in physics and chemistry led to the development of tools for doctors to investigate the body: the stethoscope to listen to the chest, the otoscope to examine ears, the ophthalmoscope to look into the eyes. Combining these developments, statistically oriented clinical observation replaced speculation and inference. Illnesses were now seen as organic lesions and patients were 'cases' of specific diseases, as the classification of diseases developed. The role of the doctor shifted from prognosis to diagnosis.

Laboratory medicine

Technological advances in the twentieth century allowed increasingly invasive investigation of organs, tissues and finally cells. The patient was seen as a cell complex, a challenge for laboratory scientists to understand and explain. The focus of diagnosis and decisions shifted from the hospital ward to the laboratory as illness was seen as a biological process. The doctor's role was now focused on the analysis of information and, as result, the explanation of what was wrong.

Loss of the holistic view

The focus on distinct, single processes has been called a *reductionist* view, as opposed to a *holistic* view that tries to conceptualize and understand the whole of a complex system. However, you should beware of simplifications – there have always been trends in medicine towards a reappearance of the holistic approach, for example seeing illness in terms of constitutional disorders (endocrine dysfunction, allergy). Another example is the recent development of neuroimmunology, which investigates the complex interactions between the central nervous system and the immune system. Generally, the awareness of social and behavioural factors in medicine and in health services is increasing. A holistic approach is essential to health and, as you will see, particularly to primary care.

 Activity 5.1

The loss of the holistic view in modern medicine may also explain the demand for alternative therapies. In the previous chapter you explored attitudes towards traditional healers. Now think of the *approach* they use and contrast it to western medicine. Are there, besides the paradigm of western medicine, any other medical paradigms in your country, which may have preserved the holistic approach to illness? Make brief notes as to any contrasting approaches you may have thought of.

 Feedback

Many of the traditional medical systems appear to be based on a holistic approach, as are animist healers and the traditional medicine in India or China. Despite the many unproven therapies, these systems have maintained their attractiveness to patients. For example, in India traditional medicine is supported by government and it has been argued that traditional medical practitioners are closer to people's own perception of health than is western medicine (Ramesh and Hyma 1996). You may also have identified schools of thought which evolved in response to modern medicine, such as anthroposophic medicine or psychosomatic medicine – these have refocused on illness as a process affecting the whole person.

Dangers of the biomedical/clinical paradigm

As a manager or as a researcher you need to rely on current disease classification, despite the fact that medical knowledge is conditional. You need also to be aware that acceptance of established knowledge has a danger of restricting and limiting useful new ideas and it can be extremely difficult to challenge established views.

 Activity 5.2

This activity invites you to explore the potential dangers of depending on hospital clinicians' knowledge of disease. Write brief notes on what those dangers might be, then compare your notes with the feedback below.

 Feedback

Some of the inherent dangers are:

1 Hospital clinicians only observe the diseased, so they may be unaware of the existence of people with similar symptoms who are not seeking care. For example, most people with chest pain seen by a cardiologist will have heart disease, yet a general practitioner may see many others with chest pain and not refer them because the pain originates from other causes.

2 Observations are confined to the clinical setting. The environment itself might induce ill health. For example, some people will have a raised blood pressure in hospital because they find the setting stressful, so-called 'white-coat' hypertension.

3 Clinicians are unable to assess factors outside the individual that may be contributing to a patient's ill health such as their job or their housing.

4 Clinicians inadvertently teach their patients to adhere to established categories of disease. The dangers of complicity between clinicians and patients have long been recognized (Englehardt and Tristram 1981):

> theories tell clinicians what to look for, what to ignore, and to act upon. Of course, they also tell patients what to see, for patients are schooled both directly and indirectly in the realities of illness and of medical disorders. As a result, given different background assumptions, different things will stand out in the patient's experience of his or her illness. In short, prevailing biomedical viewpoints fashion the life-world of patients so that their disorders appear already shaped in part by the scientific understandings of disease.

5 Clinicians may be reluctant to challenge established views. This was succinctly described by Richard Asher (1972), a British doctor, in a warning to young trainee doctors:

> We refrain from speaking about things that we observe when they are not listed in the official phenomena of the text-book description; apart from that we refrain from speaking our own opinions when they conflict too violently with generally accepted thought, or when they are greatly at variance with the opinions of those we fear. It is probably to our advantage that we do so, but it is of no advantage to the forward march of medical science.

Given these limitations, the contribution of clinicians to understanding health and disease is inevitably limited. However, that doesn't mean it is unimportant. It is a key source of hypotheses (or new ideas). Generally, clinical research takes two forms:

- the *case study* – detection of the odd, unusual or rare observation
- the *case series* – identification of common, recurring associations.

The skills required for detecting associations in a series of cases are much greater than those required for identifying single, odd events. It has been likened to the difference between noticing a very rare bird in your garden (case study) and noticing twice as many of a common bird that is a frequent visitor to your garden (case series). Most of us would manage the former but only the more observant would spot the latter.

Summary

The concept of a medical paradigm takes account of all aspects (the discourse) of medicine at a given time. Two major shifts have occurred in the western medical paradigm: from bedside medicine to hospital medicine and thence to laboratory medicine. Along with these shifts, the changing conceptualization of illness from a psychosomatic disturbance to a biochemical process has changed the relationship between sick individuals and health care practitioners. Western medicine shifted from a holistic to a reductionist perspective. However, the reappearance of the holistic approach and an increased awareness of the social and behavioural views of illness are important aspects of the current debate on health services. This chapter has concluded by considering the strengths and limitations of the methods that clinicians use in formulating medical knowledge. There is a need to question basic assumptions about any diseased state and disease categorization before considering detailed analyses or policy decisions. You should always first ask whether you can accept the implicit assumptions that are being made.

References

Asher R (1972) *Talking Sense*. London: Pitman Medical.

Englehardt JR, Tristram H (1981) Clinical judgement. *Metamedicine* 2: 301–17.

Foucault M (1981) *Madness and Civilisation: A History of Insanity in the Age of Reason*. London: Tavistock.

Jewson N (1976) The disappearance of the sick man from the medical cosmology 1770–1870. *Sociology* 10: 225–44.

Ramesh A, Hyma B (1981) Traditional Indian medicine in practice in an Indian metropolitan city. *Social Science & Medicine* 15: 69–81.

6 Staff: the challenge of professionalism

Overview

In the previous two chapters you have seen that medical knowledge is an important determinant of the key input to health services, patients. You have seen how knowledge is generated and how its basis has shifted with changes in medical paradigms. You will now explore a second key input to health services, staff, and in particular the challenge represented by the professional status of some key staff groups. You will first consider what a profession is, what distinguishes it from other occupations and how the medical profession has come to dominate in health care. Case studies will enable you to compare differences in professional development between doctors and nurses, and how practitioners from different medical systems coexist. You will then learn about the different sociological views on professional autonomy and, finally, you will consider the challenges health care professions are currently facing.

Learning objectives

After working through this chapter, you will be better able to:

- outline an 'ideal type' model of professions
- identify factors contributing to the power of professions
- compare and contrast nursing and medicine as professions
- describe how professionals from different medical paradigms coexist
- conceptualize different views on professional autonomy and identify factors challenging professional status.

Key terms

Ambulatory care Health care provided to patients without admitting them to hospital, such as general practice, outpatient clinics and day care.

Ideal type A hypothetical model of a complex real phenomenon which emphasizes its most salient features.

Ideology A set of beliefs, values and attitudes used to justify and legitimize power.

Power The ability to influence, and in particular to control, others, events and resources.

Profession An occupation based on specified knowledge and training and regulated standards of performance.

Professionalization A process whereby an occupation achieves the more independent status of a profession.

Syndicalism A militant trade union movement aimed at transferring the control and ownership of the means of production to unions.

Why study professions?

You saw in Chapter 5 how medicine has gained its status through the ability to determine the discourse on illness. But how have the main actors, the doctors, achieved their dominating status in health care? And why is it important to study professional development of health care occupations?

The concept of 'profession' is central to understanding the relationship of the different actors in health services. It provides insight into the relationship between health workers and the public. Understanding these relationships is essential to management. For example, managers need to be aware of the influence of professional groups and organizations and to be able to anticipate their resistance to change.

What is a profession?

In a colloquial sense, any kind of occupation may be regarded as a profession. But sociologists define the term 'profession' differently.

In 1947 the German sociologist, Max Weber, suggested the concept of the 'ideal type', an abstract model of a complex real phenomenon which highlights its most salient features. Note that 'ideal' is not meant in the sense of desirable (or normative) but in the sense of a pure, abstract construct. An ideal type description of a profession would have the following characteristics:

- a *'craft' tradition* – a specific body of knowledge and skills, requiring an advanced training
- a *syndicalist mode of interest representation* – similar to trade unions but with ambitions to gain control of the means of production
- a *code of ethics* – peer control through a strict code of rules
- *legal monopoly* – government regulates entry to the profession by law and specifies requirements for training and qualifications, thereby restricting activities of other occupations in the field
- *ideological monopoly* – a means of enabling the profession to dominate the views on its subject and to make it widely accepted. These are the values, attitudes and beliefs underlying a profession's way of achieving and maintaining privileged status. Ideology is used to justify and legitimize professional status and gives its members a sense of importance and cohesiveness. Professional ideology has evolved over time and during this process the views held by the profession have also become shared and internalized by the public.

You can use the ideal type description of a profession to contrast professional status of different occupations or to compare the process of professionalization in different countries.

The combination of these factors produces the privileged status of professions in society. Their status relative to other occupations can be assessed by:

- *wealth* – higher income, as a result of a better position in the marketplace
- *prestige* – the esteem in which the group is held by others
- *power* – the ability to influence decisions and other occupations in the field.

Activity 6.1

Using the ideal type description, identify and list examples of occupations that have achieved professional status in your country.

Feedback

You are likely to have listed law and medicine in the first instance, followed perhaps by occupations such as dentistry, architecture, accountancy, teaching and nursing. The extent of professionalization of the latter professions varies between countries. The first established professionals were self-employed and charged fees. Their members were granted a privileged status through government regulation. In most countries professionalization is an ongoing process, with a number of occupations trying to professionalize themselves by forming associations and striving to establish recognition for ethical standards, formalized training and specialized knowledge. However, few have achieved professional status and probably none has achieved professional status as complete as that accorded to law and medicine.

The power of professions

Having explored the characteristics of professions in general, you will now examine in more detail the basis of power of the medical profession. Historically, the rise of the medical profession was related to achieving a legal and ideological monopoly. Factors facilitating this process include the scientific background of medical knowledge and organized education.

Power is a sociological and political concept that is key to understanding the behaviour of social systems. In Chapter 5 you learned about the relationship between language and power. Power is the ability to influence, or in Weber's definition, to control others, events and resources. Power can be *coercive* by using force, or based on *authority* which is accepted by others and seen as legitimate. There are also more subtle forms of power, for instance the *power of non-decision-making* and, as you have seen earlier, the power to shape the beliefs and values of others. The following activity invites you to reflect on the power of doctors in health services.

Activity 6.2

As you have seen, Professional power is based on:

- technical expertise
- authority
- Clientele
- uncertainty
- relationship to other professions

Suggest an example of each as it relates to doctors.

Feedback

Compare your explanations with those in the completed Table 6.1. Are they broadly comparable?

Table 6.1 Key aspects of professional power

Professional power is based on	Example relating to doctors
technical expertise	Scientific background of medical knowledge, special skills, for example surgical operations
authority	Doctors provide a widely acknowledged view on health and illness; they are accepted as persons to give ultimate advice in health matters
clientele	Unlike many other occupations, doctors have individual clients (patients), who engage in a personal relationship based on trust
uncertainty	The uncertainty of need for health care and of the outcomes of care lead people to seek professional advice from experts
relationship to other professions	Medicine has developed as the lead profession in health services, for example doctors are better paid and occupy higher ranks in the hierarchy than other health workers

Comparison of medicine and nursing

The following is an extract from a 1990 book by Phil Strong, a sociologist, and Jane Robinson, a nurse, that will give you a good insight into the differences of professional status between doctors and nurses. Though the text refers to a particular situation in the UK in the late 1980s, the interviews provide an insight into some universal problems of the power relations between different groups of health workers. Doctors and nurses were being asked to take more control over the management of resources and greater responsibility for many of the day-to-day management processes.

Activity 6.3

 Doctors and nurses

If managers' main problem with medicine was its rampant individualism, many of their problems with nursing were quite the reverse. While medical syndicalism was the exemplar of the potential power of a profession, nursing was organized on quite opposite principles. Yet despite this fundamental difference, the principles on which nursing was based still created huge problems for management. Where doctors exhibited an excess of individual initiative, too often nurses had no initiative at all. For all the attempts to create something closer to a profession, many managers still felt that key aspects of nursing were dominated by an outlandish sense of hierarchy. A quasi-military discipline could extend throughout nursing, to every level of the organization:

> Nurses took the wrong turn at the very start of nurse management. They should have taken the professional role. What we need is nurse practitioners equivalent to the hospital consultant who, like doctors, would have peers. They could be managed either by nurses or non-nurses. But, instead, nursing got trapped in the strange blind alley of a hierarchical system where to get any money you had to go up the bureaucracy. But nurses are basically staff, not line. (District medical officer)

> [It's being] afraid of failing. That's what I think is the biggest thing with nursing staff. They are so used to being criticized if they lose a pill or somebody has happened to miscount them – and then they have to report it. And they are so used to being told, 'How could you let that happen, nurse?' (Senior nurse)

Moreover, although there was a radical internal reform movement within nursing – led by the Royal College – to create a proper nursing profession, comparatively modest attempts at professional development could still meet considerable opposition, not just from outsiders elsewhere in the service, but from senior figures within its own ranks. Many nurse managers, so it was held, positively enjoyed bossing their subordinates and had little interest in actively soliciting their junior staff's opinion or seriously enhancing their technical skills. To do so was too threatening to their own status:

> Most senior nurses are so concerned to deliver nursing services that they don't think how to develop nursing. Perhaps it's because they're so hierarchical and insecure. It's a particular style of management. (Senior nurse)

This hierarchical world could extend, so it was argued, deep into some nurses' private lives and personality. In those parts of the country with expensive housing, the closure and sale of nurses' accommodation presented major problems in retaining staff. None the less, some managers were glad to see the old nurses' homes abolished. Nurses who had lived there for years could become institutionalized, as could those who worked too long in the same place.

All these factors, so managers held, had a further consequence which distinguished nursing quite dramatically from medicine. The elaborate hierarchy, the lack of any developed sense of professional identity and the initiation into submission from the earliest years meant that nursing was extraordinarily weak in the face of external opposition. Nursing might be huge in number, but there was relatively little occupational solidarity . . . As a result, where nurses often found it hard to oppose the new management, chief executives had to proceed much more gingerly with doctors:

> All too often in nursing, you start out with the support of your colleagues and when you get to the chairman's door and knock on it and say, 'We're all saying, "No!" ' you suddenly find there's no one with you! (Senior nurse)

> The capacity of nurses to screw the system is much less than that of doctors. (Chief executive)

Finally, some nurse managers noted that although nursing possessed its own elaborate hierarchy which stretched, since 1974, through every management tier, its place at the highest levels was very far from secure. However formidable a senior nurse might appear to a ward sister, her position was far weaker than her colleagues' and rivals'.

There was, then, a quite extraordinary contrast in managers' eyes between the individual power of doctors and the collective feebleness of nurses; between medicine's influence at the highest levels and nursing's notional representation; between doctors' fierce syndical- ism and nursing's massive internal hierarchy. But having drawn that contrast, it is also crucial to see that the two are very intimately linked. Nursing's hierarchy stemmed not so much from within nursing itself, as from the many powerful forces – medicine, gender and the demands of an extremely labour-intensive industry – which had created, shaped and controlled the nursing trade. The effect of these three closely interlinked forces was to powerfully subordinate the entire occupation. As a consequence, it had reproduced internally the structure of its external domination. Tight control from without meant rigid hierarchy within. Though many deeply resented it, nurses had been – and mostly continued to be – the handmaidens of the medical profession, a servant class . . . Even the most senior nurses could be patronized – or bullied – by some members of the medical profession. The following speaker recounted her arrival eight years previously at one of Britain's more famous teaching hospitals:

> Within a fortnight I was summoned by the medical executive committee to account for my being appointed. So I went before them. I had to wait for twenty minutes and the person who went in before me was the Director of Nursing Services for the acute hospital and she was just berated. They were incredibly rude. She was reduced to a quivering wreck. It was obviously a common practice in the past to call matron to account . . . They felt they had every right to ask me to account for yet another post in nursing administration and just what was I doing . . . I was there three-quarters of an hour and they berated me one after another – things like, 'We don't want American- style academic nurses coming here' . . . though *afterwards* one or two individual consult- ants came up and wished me good luck. (Senior nurse)

Managers, in their turn, might simply reflect medical attitudes. Doctors were the real bosses and their values could permeate the entire organization, affecting the new manage- ment quite as much as the old . . . Most doctors and health care managers were, of course, male, most nurses female. Such institutional stratification was regularly reinforced, so some female nurse managers reported, in their interaction with other staff:

> My appointment to the local medical committee was for six months in the first instance. When that six months was up I raised the matter as no one else had and offered to leave the room while they discussed it. They said there was no need and the chairman made the typical remark which you learn to ignore that they had to keep me on as I was prettier than the rest. (Nurse manager)

Our aim . . . has been to capture a few simple stereotypes of the clinical trades, to distil service managers' views of the worst organizational attributes of medicine and nursing – the features that made radical reform so essential in their eyes. In the crude model presented here, the two trades had a strange symmetry, each being a bizarre reverse image of the other. Doctors were men and nurses were women. Doctors were small in number but possessed extraordinary power. Nursing was vast in size but amazingly weak in influence. Doctors were educated and nurses were ignorant. Doctors were wealthy and nurses were poorly paid. Medicine had a vast scientific base, nursing had hardly any. Doctors were independent professionals, possessing a fierce autonomy in their clinical judgement; nursing was not a profession and was notorious for its hierarchy, indeed, for an almost military discipline. Doctors were famed for their solidarity when threatened, nurses renowned for the ease with which they gave way. Doctors were to be skilful, nurses were to be virtuous.

 Feedback

1 The text gives a variety of reasons for differences in professional development between doctors and nurses, for example:

- lack of independence – nurses are more bound by hierarchy and quasi-military discipline
- lack of autonomy in clinical judgement
- lack of own scientific knowledge and language
- lack of solidarity and syndicalist mode of interest representation
- lack of influence on decision making.

Note also that many of the problems are related to the traditional gender role of women in society: nursing is often viewed as women's work and seen as a domestic service which does not require expert knowledge.

2 The status of nursing varies internationally and so do requirements for training, career prospects and payment levels relative to doctors. Different curricula and job entry requirements may even exist within a country between ambulatory care and hospitals. The nurse–doctor ratio varies widely (see Chapter 17) and this is, to some extent, also a reflection of the professional status of nurses. Academically trained nurses are more prevalent in the English-speaking world and in Nordic countries.

Strengthening nursing education and professional development is high on the agenda of many countries. Where independent nurse practitioners have been introduced, this has often been seen as a challenge to the medical profession.

Medical systems

In all countries, doctors have had to negotiate their relationship with practitioners who subscribe to another system of medical thought such as acupuncture or homeopathy. In some countries, biomedical doctors (sometimes referred to as allopathic) have come to dominate through fairly ruthless measures aimed at controlling and suppressing other systems. However, in many countries an accommodation has been reached in which the different roles and contributions of various practitioners have been respected.

 Activity 6.4

The following is an extract from a book written in the late 1980s by Murray Last, an anthropologist (Last 1996). As you read it, make notes on the following issues:

1 The contrasting ways in which India, China and what is referred to as the Third World model have sought to integrate western and traditional, indigenous medical systems.
2 The source of legitimacy of practitioners.

 Integrated systems: Asian pluralism

Under British imperial legislation, Indian practitioners of Ayurvedic, Siddha, and Unani medicine were at liberty not only to practice but to develop associations and schools of medicine. For nearly a century these alternative medical institutions have developed to rival those set up for 'cosmopolitan' (or 'Western') medicine by the imperial regime. All the formal trappings of professionalism – theoretical texts for teaching in university courses, research institutes, an autonomous governing council with statutory powers, hospitals, state funding, a specialized drug industry – have long been in place. Nonetheless, since independence the government of India has built up the 'cosmopolitan,' hospital-based services, not only supporting a strong medical profession with qualifications that met international standards but also developing a network of rural dispensaries and related services to such an extent that use of 'Western' medicine is reported to be as widespread as Ayurveda. Not merely is it now as widely available, but it is offered at lower cost. In this situation, Ayurvedic colleges are said to be having difficulties recruiting applicants of comparable caliber. Homeopathy, with an origin that links it theoretically with Islamic medicine, has been adopted and adapted, particularly in Bengal, as an Indian system of medicine and similarly given rise to formal professional structures.

Other, less systematic therapeutic systems survive without professionalization on the margins of the national medical culture and meeting specific needs the various formal systems cannot adequately provide for. Many are religious in essence, using temples or festivals as focal points for healing and relying on charity rather than government or local state funds.

Legal models like India's are widespread in south and east Asia, with professional recognition given to more than one system of medicine. In recent years the more restrictive legislation carried over from the colonial period has been replaced, in part as a response to nationalist feeling, in part to make the law match social reality. The degree to which all formally recognized medical professions are run as bureaucracies by the state depends on the local political matrix. India, with its open, democratic system, reflects that political tradition in its attitudes to medical politics and so leaves practitioners largely to regulate themselves. China, by contrast, being Marxist in ideology, has always recognized Chinese traditional medicine in all its variety but integrated it into the state-run services. 'Barefoot doctors' were one solution to the problem of integration; trained partly in traditional and mainly in 'Western' medicine, they served as medical auxiliaries. Another solution was to maintain state-financed hospitals in which acupuncture, moxibustion and herbal therapy were available as required.

. . . These two systems – Indian and Chinese – have provided models for incorporating indigenous practitioners elsewhere, but there are questions as to their appropriateness, particularly in Africa, where, historically, centralized states have tended not to create elaborate medical bureaucracies, with ancient written texts and systematic theorization. Furthermore, in both India and China there was considerable unity to the medical traditions, which had largely ceased to be as culture or region specific as are many such traditions in Africa.

A final model which *de facto* (if not *de jure*) is integrative is to be found in Third World countries whose economic resources and colonial history have left them with the legacy of small, secondary professions not powerful enough to effect a monopoly. Although their legal traditions and the current political matrix may differ, these differences may count for less than the characteristics they have in common.

The characteristics of the Third World model are (1) a relatively weak and underfinanced system of hospital medicine, largely urban centered, staffed by doctors (nationals and foreigners) trained to different standards and routines in a number of different countries; (2) a legal system that privileges that hospital system yet is unable, in practical terms, to outlaw any alternative; (3) a very large number of local practitioners of traditional medicine, bonesetters, midwives, barber-surgeons, and so forth who have always tried to meet the health needs of the community; (4) a wide spectrum of modern alternative therapies, alongside a market in medical drugs imported, sometimes unmarked and instructionless, from all over the world; and (5) a population that is dispersed and often difficult of access yet has high rates of morbidity and mortality.

. . . Seen from below, . . . the legitimacy of a healing system is quite distinct from the kind of political legality so far discussed. This grass-roots legitimacy may arise, as Weber suggests, either from the community's own traditions or from the healer's personal charisma. Whatever the source, at this level it is clinical practice, not political philosophy, that is determinant. At the core of clinical practice is the therapeutic triangle of relationships of patient, healer, and a local public that includes both kin and others in the community. The structure of these relationships and the medical concepts that inform them vary widely within any country today, indeed even within communities. But taken together, the distinct patterns of relationships and concepts rendered visible in this therapeutic triangle constitute the various separate medical subcultures that, for convenience, we can label as Ayurveda, for example, or homeopathy. Constituting more diffuse a subculture are those individual practitioners whose therapies we generally categorize together under the heading 'traditional medicine.'

Professionalization of this traditionally diffuse subculture seeks to give it not only a certain political unity but also at the community level a coherent image, akin to a successful trademark with its associated goodwill, that would guarantee a uniformly high quality of service. Contemporary sociological analyses are obsessed with the power of professions as interest groups within society at large, whereas earlier analysts were intrigued by the way ethical rather than commercial norms were (in theory at least) established and enforced, by the way too that unethical or incompetent practitioners were controlled. Unfashionable though these concerns may be (or simply taken for granted), nonetheless for patients at the clinical level these concerns are central. The legality of a practice is less important than the practitioner's moral standing or trustworthiness. Where a community and its practitioners have worked together for years, this local legitimation is rarely problematic. Elsewhere, and particularly in towns, where practitioners or patients may be newcomers, initial legitimation of this kind might potentially come from professional membership.

In short, a professionalization from below has always existed in some form or other in long-established communities. The question is how to expand it to meet modem circumstances. Is politically orientated professionalization from above compatible with socially sanctioned professionalization from below? A major difference between the two perspectives on professionalization lies in the ways professional knowledge is perceived (whether bureaucratically from above or clinically from below) and what the relationship is between the two.

 Feedback

I India recognized more than one medical system. Practitioners of all systems were at liberty to practise and form professional associations. This was partly driven by social reality and partly a response to nationalist feelings. Professions were encouraged to develop self-regulation.

In China, the Maoist state actively sought to integrate traditional medicine with western medicine. Barefoot doctors were trained not only in western medicine but also in acupuncture, herbal therapy and other systems. Hospitals made use of all available systems.

The Third World model accepts its inability to control the various local practitioners due to the lack of a strong system of western medicine and, therefore, people's dependence on indigenous systems.

2 Legitimacy of practitioners and medical systems is derived from the local community's own traditions or the personal charisma of practitioners. This is essentially a pragmatic, experiential approach rather than one based on political philosophy.

The role of the medical profession in society

Does the public benefit from having independent professions or not? This is a much debated issue and you will look at it by examining the different public views held on the role of the medical profession. The following paragraphs (based on Moore 1994) outline briefly some of the views held by social scientists on the autonomy of the medical profession.

The longest established view was that advanced by the American sociologist, Talcott Parsons (1902–79), in 1939. His *functionalist* view welcomed the notion of professions, seeing the legitimation of professional status as a means of protecting patients from harm. Patients accept the authority of doctors. They trust doctors and expect them to have the highest competence. Therefore knowledge and skills need to be guaranteed by educational standards. To protect the intimate relationship between doctors and patients, the profession needs to be granted an autonomous status, independent from state interference. Professionalism is thought to allow a more flexible response to patients' needs than tightly controlled health services. As only doctors can judge their peers, they need to have the right to discipline members who violate the code of conduct. Thus professionalism plays a beneficial role by serving both the needs of the individual and of society.

In contrast, there have been several critiques that challenge Parsons' view. In the *Marxist* view, professions are considered a middle-class privilege, mystifying and stabilizing the power of the ruling class. This was seen as part of a wider struggle between classes for economic, social and political advantages, a struggle that was limited by the mode of production.

An alternative critique propounded by Elliot Freidson in 1974 emphasized the role of *self-interest* in the formation of professions. To him, professionalization is similar to trade unionism, a way of increasing the rewards for labour. Doctors have been particularly successful in eliminating their competitors and creating a monopoly. They have managed to keep remuneration high through market closure. And in due course, they have managed to convey the image that only members of the profession can provide services properly. In this view, professionalism is beneficial only at the expense of other occupations and to members who pursue their own interests. This view partly echoed the concerns of the liberal Irish playwright, George Bernard Shaw, in 1911 who suggested that 'All professions are conspiracies against the laity.'

More recently, the Austrian theologian Ivan Illich (1974) criticized professionalism as a way of colonizing other sectors of social life (medical imperialism) and disguising the fact that doctors produce ill health (iatrogenesis). In his view, professionalism does more harm than good. Doctors don't just provide health services but attempt to take control over other aspects of life. Examples of medical expansion include the *medicalization* of childbirth, disabilities, problems of ageing and death. An increasing number of social problems have been handed over to the medical profession, thereby extending its authority to define what is good or wrong and barring other professions and lay people from dealing with health problems. Medical expansion is seen as a threat as it weakens individual abilities to cope with illness and hides away pain and death, which are natural parts of life.

Activity 6.5

Based on what you have just read.

1 Write down four key arguments in favour of and four against independent status of doctors.
2 Contrast briefly the different views and compare them with your own experience in health services.
3 In your opinion, which view best matches the role of the medical profession?

 Feedback

1 Some of the arguments for and against professional autonomy that you may have are identified are listed in Table 6.2.

Table 6.2 Arguments for and against professional autonomy

For	Against
Trust	Middle class monopoly
Defence of individual	Medical expansion
Peer control	Dominated by self-interest
Flexibility	Lack of accountability

2 Though medical expansion has clearly occurred, Illich's generalizing view of the role of experts has been criticized as exaggerated and misleading (Strong 1979). On the other hand, the functionalist view, which had developed among the early writers, appears to be naive in not taking account of the self-interest of the medical profession. Friedson's view has incorporated the aspect of self-interest and given an explanation of professional power, which has been widely acknowledged.

3 Obviously your answer will depend on the professional status of doctors in your country. Opinions on professional status have changed over time, as has the power of the profession. Some recent publications on the subject have been less critical than those of the 1970s and 1980s (Cruess and Cruess 1997).

Do professions have a future?

As you have seen, professional status is not an inherent right – it is granted by society. The maintenance of the professional status accorded to doctors depends on the public's belief that doctors are trustworthy. Has the perception of the public changed? Has the medical profession lost power relative to other actors in health services?

Activity 6.6

Think of the status and power of doctors in your country.

- Has it changed in recent years?
- What challenges have there been to medical knowledge?
- Have challenges been mounted by other professionals working in health care?

Make brief notes in response to these questions, referring to your own experience and to examples from this and previous chapters.

 Feedback

You are more than likely to have noted that the status and power of doctors has changed in recent years. These changes, which represent threats to traditional medical interests, can also be seen as opportunities for changing the way health services are conceived and delivered.

1 *Managerialism* – the growing importance of managers and management processes in health care. Decisions on resource allocation are no longer left to professional autonomy. Doctors are being made increasingly accountable to those paying for health services. (See the article by Relman in Chapter 2.)

2 *Lay knowledge and self-help movements* – consumers have become better informed and may develop into experts in dealing with particular health problems, thereby challenging professional knowledge (see Chapter 10).

3 *Boundary disputes* – while there is medical expansion there are also challenges from other professions taking over tasks formerly performed by doctors. For example, think of the increasing number of medicines sold without prescription by pharmacists. Nurse practitioners performing tasks formerly reserved to doctors are often seen as challenge. Think also of psychologists or social workers dealing with drug addicts who, it was once thought, should be exclusively treated by doctors.

4 *Medical pluralism* – the profession is increasingly divided. The interests of doctors in primary care may conflict with those in secondary and tertiary care. Subgroups within the profession challenge traditional views. Growing specialization makes it difficult to represent the interests of all doctors. For example, in many countries instead of a single organization representing all surgeons, there are several subspecialties with potentially opposing views.

5 *Effectiveness in question* – the issue of the extent to which medical interventions are effective has gained public attention. Many treatments have only little effect on outcomes but are promoted with professional authority. The public is increasingly aware of the limits of medicine and is becoming more critical towards medical knowledge.

6 *Ideological opposition* – doctors face opposition from other groups in society, such as other professions, social movements or parties who try to challenge the ideological monopoly of the profession. Examples include social movements fighting for consumer

rights in medicine, feminist groups challenging the role of medicine in childbirth, and religious groups challenging the medical definition of death and criteria for organ transplantation.

7 More general problems are those of a *loss of faith* in experts and public institutions and the *contracting role of the state*, which in some countries is taking less responsibility for health care and for protecting professional status.

These challenges do not mean that professionalism has no future or that its power is necessarily declining. There are, however, visible signs of decline in many countries. For example, in a number of countries recent health care reforms have been decided without the consent of the medical profession. Much of the future role of the medical profession depends on its ability to respond to these challenges. Professional organizations are increasingly aware that they need to meet the expectations of the public in order to remain trustworthy (a theme you return to in Chapter 19). And obviously they will meet these expectations more easily by placing the objective of serving the public over self-interest.

Summary

Professionalism is a key concept in explaining the role of some key occupations in health services and in society. Professional status is based on formalized training and knowledge, peer control and a legal and ideological monopoly. The state plays an important role in granting and protecting professional status. There are significant differences in professional development, internationally and between professional groups within health services. In this chapter you have considered the context of professional power and examined the different views held on professional autonomy. Finally, you have reviewed the changes in professional status and the challenges that professions currently face.

References

Cruess SR, Cruess RL (1997) Professionalism must be taught. *British Medical Journal* 315: 1674–5.

Freidson E (1974) *Profession of Medicine*. Chicago: University of Chicago Press.

Illich I (1974) *Medical Nemesis*. London: Bantam Books.

Last M (1996) The professionalisation of indigenous healers, in C Sergent, T Johnson (eds) *Medical Anthropology: Contemporary Theory and Method*. Westport, CT: Praeger.

Moore S (1994) *A Level Sociology*. London: Letts Educational.

Parsons T (1939) The professions and social structure. *Social Forum* 17: 457–67.

Strong PM (1979) Sociological imperialism and the profession of medicine. *Social Science & Medicine* 13: 199–215.

Strong PM, Robinson J (1990) *The NHS. Under New Management*. Milton Keynes: Open University Press.

Weber M (1947) *Theory of Social and Economic Organization*. Glencoe, IL: Free Press.

7 Funding health care

Overview

In the previous three chapters you explored two key inputs to health care: patients and staff. You will now explore the other important input, finance. This chapter explains the principal sources of finance and the challenges in allocating those funds in publicly funded systems.

Learning objectives

After working through this chapter, you will be better able to:

- **describe the difficulties in interpreting international differences in expenditure**
- **describe the main objectives of a funding system**
- **distinguish between the principal ways of funding health care through taxes, social insurance and private payments.**

Key terms

Allocative (economic, Pareto, social) efficiency A situation in which it is not possible to improve the welfare of one person in an economy without making someone else worse off.

Capitation payments A prospective means of paying health care staff based on the number of people they provide care for.

Co-payments (user fees) Direct payments made by users of health services as a contribution to their cost (e.g. prescription charges).

Fee-for-service A means of paying health care staff on the basis of the actual items of care provided.

Gross domestic product (GDP) The market value of the goods and services produced within the borders of a country (consumption plus investment plus government purchases plus net exports).

Not-for-profit organizations Organizations with no shareholders, so all income received for providing services is paid to staff or invested in improving the organization.

Technical (operational, productive) efficiency Using only the minimum necessary resources to finance, purchase and deliver a particular activity or set of activities (i.e. avoiding waste).

International differences in health care expenditure

As you are aware, funding levels vary between countries. The amount spent on health care depends on wealth – there is a strong correlation between the proportion of gross domestic product (GDP) spent on health and the wealth of the country (less than 3% in low income countries, 9–13% in the richest ones; see Table 7.1). In this sense health care behaves like a luxury good – more is bought at high incomes.

Table 7.1 International comparison of health care expenditure (1997–2000) and provision of physicians and hospital beds (1995–2000)

Country	% GDP (1997–2000)	% public funding (1997–2000)	US$ per capita (1997–2000)	Physicians per 1 000 people (1995–2000)	Beds per 1 000 people (1995–2000)
Azerbaijan	0.9	75	8	3.6	8.6
DR Congo	1.5	74	9	0.1	NA
Ecuador	2.4	50	26	1.7	1.6
Indonesia	2.7	24	19	NA	NA
N Korea	2.1	77	18	3.0	NA
Nigeria	2.2	21	8	NA	NA
Romania	2.9	64	48	1.8	7.6
Cameroon	4.3	25	24	0.1	NA
Russia	5.3	73	92	4.2	12.1
Poland	6.0	70	246	2.2	4.9
S Korea	6.0	44	584	1.3	6.1
UK	7.3	81	1 747	1.8	4.1
Canada	9.1	72	2 058	2.1	3.9
France	9.5	76	2 057	3.0	8.2
Germany	10.6	75	2 422	3.6	9.1
USA	13.0	44	4 499	2.8	3.6

NA = not available
GDP = gross domestic product

Source: data extracted from WHO website.

 Activity 7.1

Why are meaningful comparisons of how much a country spends on health care so difficult?

 Feedback

First, it is not clear what should be included. There is no clear line between health and spending on other types of social care. Second, exchange rates may not reflect the value of money in terms of services provided and the fact that drug prices tend to be in US dollars causes further distortions. For example, although only US$19 is spent per capita in Indonesia, one dollar will buy more physician time than it will in France or Canada.

Objectives when funding health care

Fundamentally, financing of health services should ensure:

- that all people who need care have access to health services (*equity*)
- that services are provided in a way that provides best value for money (*efficiency*).

But what inputs should be provided in what quantities? Obviously no health system can provide every kind of service in any desired quantity. All inputs need to be paid for and covered by the funds available. Any funding system should:

- be acceptable to the population covered
- make clear the mechanisms of funding and the associated entitlements
- be adequate
- be sustainable
- spend as little as possible on collecting funds
- be congruent with health care priorities, such as achieving social equity.

Given that some of these are not absolute (e.g. acceptability to the population) but will vary from country to country, it is inevitable that there is no universal solution for all countries.

Sources of finance

Reasons for departure from direct payment (that applies to most non-health products and services) include market failure (i.e. problems of missing or asymmetric information distort the workings of the market) and equity. Many people argue that access to effective health care should not be dependent on ability to pay. As a result, a number of different approaches have developed over the past 250 years. The approaches fall into two categories:

- those based on solidarity (mutual support). The main solidarity systems are *social health insurance* and *taxation*. In both cases the principle is that contributions are made on the basis of ability to pay (somehow defined) and access to care is based on need (also somehow defined).
- those where actual or expected payments are based on use of services. The three main sources of funds not dependent on solidarity are *actuarial* or *private insurance*, *medical savings accounts* and *direct payment* by individual patients.

Almost all countries use a mixture of approaches and no approach really works the way it is planned to work. There are elements of solidarity in apparently actuarial systems and many of the equity objectives in tax and social insurance are not achieved. Despite that, it is important to understand the pros and cons of the options available.

Tax and social insurance

It is sometimes argued that there is little difference between funding from tax and social insurance – in both cases people make compulsory income-related contributions and gain access to care on the basis of need. In some countries social insurance is operated like a tax and is under the control of government. Some tax systems started as social insurance but the distinction between compulsory contributions and taxes gradually disappeared. In other countries the social insurance fund (or funds) operates with a high degree of independence from government and effectively turns every patient into a private patient.

The most common base for tax or social insurance is income from employment. Where most incomes are derived from employment this may be a good proxy for total income. However, both now and even more so in the future, there are reasons to be concerned about how well this will reflect ability to pay. The proportion of people in long term employment with large employers is low in middle income and poor countries, and is falling in most countries. More people are employed in small organizations, more are self-employed, more are working on contract, and more are on pensions and other non-employment income. Widening disparities of wealth make employment income a poor proxy for ability to pay. Other disadvantages of social insurance are that it is expensive to assess wealth whereas salaries and wages are easy to calculate and assess, and a sudden increase in the level of unemployment will lead to a concomitant fall in funds available for health care.

Actuarial or private insurance

Actuarial insurance assesses the risk of a person needing treatment and charges a premium based on this risk. Given the distribution of risk in the population, this means that the actuarially fair premium is higher for older, poorer and visibly less well people. In practice, assessing risk is expensive and so insurance companies normally do not calculate risk for each individual but determine the premium on the basis of sociodemographic characteristics and self-reported health status. The process can be jeopardized by governments which prevent some information being collected – for example, it may be illegal to ask if a potential customer is HIV positive. The high costs of collecting data may mean that some solidarity exists in (supposedly) actuarial insurance. In addition, if policies cover families there may be limited cross-subsidy. Little can be done to encourage solidarity between richer and poorer people in actuarial insurance. However, it would in principle be possible to get around the problem of variation of premiums by age. Insurance works well to share risk when events and outcomes for individuals are genuinely unknown. Contracts could in principle be taken out early in life, before any information on risk were known, and these life-long contracts could provide a mechanism for subsidy of the old by the young and of the sick by the healthy. The problem is that the contracts are normally too short to allow this to happen. Taken to the ultimate, insurance would be agreed at or prior to conception. However, with advances in genetics even this may not continue to be such a straightforward option.

Private insurance normally results in incomplete population coverage, and in general this problem is worse in poorer countries and those with more unequal income distribution. In many countries, private insurance exists in parallel with tax-funded or social insurance sources. There is considerable debate as to whether the additional funds take pressure off the public system or enjoy hidden subsidies (such as employing trained staff but not contributing to their training costs).

Medical savings accounts

Medical savings accounts, which require patients or families to save for the purpose of routine, non-catastrophic health care, have attracted widespread interest. A version has been used in Singapore for some years, and they have been suggested in the USA as a substitute for some employer-based insurance. They are based on the idea that a major problem is not the inability of families to afford health care but rather the difficulty in ensuring that the necessary funds are available at the time of need. Families or individuals have to set aside money each month, and this continues till a sufficiently large fund is established. When money is spent from the fund the family must start saving again to replenish it. In the case of Singapore the fund can be passed on to the next generation. Family funds provide limited solidarity across generations but not more generally. In Singapore the main savings account system has two schemes to subsidize poorer and sicker people, and some more general subsidies are available for hospital services, especially the more basic services.

Direct payments

Direct payment by individuals can deter use of services. The problem is that studies suggest that their deterrent effects are similar for more and less useful services. However, it is also clear that they can be an effective way of raising funds and that people prefer better quality services with higher fees to lower quality care at lower cost. Since deterrent effects are related to incomes it is possible to get round some of the problems if exemptions are allowed for poorer or chronically sick people.

✎ Activity 7.2

The different sources of finance used around the world are discussed in the following extract by three health economists, Barbara McPake, Lilani Kumaranayake and Charles Normand (2002). Once you have read it, note the characteristics of a country you are familiar with in terms of: the extent to which solidarity exists; the balance between public and private funding; the existence of 'default privatization', and the degree to which the system is segmented or integrated. You may need to obtain information from government or other sources (international bodies such as WHO or OECD) to complete this task.

📖 Health systems around the world

Health systems are typically characterised by 'insurance'. This is broadly defined to mean that users pay regularly towards health system expenses in order to avoid bills that would make an unacceptable hole in the household budget at the time of use, and in order to share risk between larger population groups so that no one family faces completely unaffordable catastrophic costs. Broadly defined, public systems can be considered a form of insurance, with the relevant share of tax effectively equivalent to a health insurance premium. More commonly, the term 'health insurance' is restricted to arrangements where separate premiums and a separate 'earmarked' fund for health services is created. Even within this narrower definition of insurance a wide variety of arrangements is found. 'Social insurance' implies compulsory membership and usually a public or quasi-public insurance agent. Private insurance is offered by private insurance companies and is usually voluntary (South Korea's private but compulsory insurance is an exception) but is, nonetheless, usually subject to substantial regulation.

There are very few cases of 'pure' health systems that are neatly captured by these archetype descriptions. Wide and increasing variation is possible within each archetype. While many countries' health systems are dominated by one or other archetype (while usually having small sub-components equivalent to one another), it is equally common for countries to have a number of important subsectors corresponding to different archetypes. Some country examples will serve to make this case.

At the extreme public end of the spectrum of archetypes, the health system of the former German Democratic Republic was centrally and publicly financed and provided, with almost all services free of charge to patients. All health staff were salaried and the private sector was extremely small. The system has now been integrated with that of the Federal German Republic. The arrangements were typical of the former Communist countries of Central and Eastern Europe that are now all undergoing substantial reform. However, in practice, divergence from the pure public model is reported in many of these countries to the extent that while intended to be free, substantial 'under-the-counter' payments seem to have been made by patients in order to secure services, a form of default privatisation. Nevertheless, this Semashko system, at least in its intended form, occupies the extreme, most publicly dominated end of the archetypal range.

The UK health system is dominated by the largely publicly provided and financed National Health Service (NHS) but includes some user charges (for example, for dental and optical services and for prescriptions) and also contains a small private insurance sector outside the NHS. Most of the resources used within the NHS are owned or employed publicly, but primary-care doctors, known as general practitioners, are contracted private individuals or firms. Further complications have been introduced by two rounds of reforms in the 1990s that have separated purchasing and providing functions (while maintaining the public character of both), and have increased the role of private investment funding in the system. Examples of other countries whose systems are dominated by public provision and finance but with more private components than the former Communist countries include Denmark (where non-hospital services are provided under public contract by private practitioners and certain co-payments exist), Sweden (where private practice is common only in occupational health and dentistry), Ireland (where richer people have more limited access to public services and voluntary but public insurance covers 30 per cent of the population) and New Zealand (where primary providers are private practitioners and a range of co-payments apply).

A number of poorer countries have modelled their health systems on either the British or the Semashko model. Taking Uganda as an example, the health system was designed to be dominated by public finance and provision. A range of publicly owned health facilities from small aid posts in most remote regions, intended to provide services for minor illnesses, through health centres, district and regional hospitals and two teaching hospitals in the two largest cities, are all publicly equipped, directly employ all health personnel, and are publicly supplied with drugs and other non-durable items. Recent reform of the system includes major decentralisation, in line with general administrative decentralisation in the country. However, problems of inadequate resources and poor management of resources in the public sector have ensured that the public system has for some time not been as dominant in health service provision as was originally intended. Within the public system, substantial 'default privatisation' is reported, as in the former Communist countries discussed above. In addition, pure private practice fills the gaps the public sector has left, and covers a high, if difficult to document, proportion of primary-care provision. This includes some of the purest private sector arrangements to be found, with unregulated providers selling unsubsidised or taxed services directly to health service users. At the hospital level private not-for-profit providers (mainly mission-run facilities) play a substantial role. Examples of countries in which similar descriptions apply include India, Pakistan, Bangladesh, Kenya, Tanzania and Ghana, although the extent of 'default privatisation' within the public system varies considerably.

'Social insurance' dominates the health systems of most of the remaining industrialised countries. The Bismarck model of social insurance, developed in Germany, has often been considered the standard model of social insurance. In the former [pre-reunification] Federal Republic of Germany 75 per cent of the population were insured compulsorily, about 13 per cent voluntarily with the same (quasi-public) statutory sickness funds while 10 per cent of the population were insured privately. (This situation has changed with the integration of the former GDR into the system.) There are both public and private providers (51 per cent of hospital beds are public; ambulatory care physicians and pharmacies are largely private). Both types mainly operate on contract to the statutory sickness funds (although investment costs are usually directly funded by state governments), and there are only minor co-payments paid by patients at the time of use. Examples of countries in which similar system models operate include Belgium (however, co-payments are much more substantial and a higher proportion of health service costs are met through tax-based finance), France (with 99 per cent insurance with statutory sickness funds but a 'reimbursement' model for many health sector transactions whereby health service users pay and are later reimbursed), the Netherlands (where recent reforms aim to stimulate competition in both the insurance and provision markets), and Austria.

The majority of Latin American countries (defined as Mexico and the countries of Central and South America, excluding the Caribbean island nations) contain three important sub-systems: public, social insurance and private (both insurance and out-of-pocket financed). Taking Peru as an example, about 30 per cent of health sector expenditure goes to public sector providers, 35 per cent to separate social insurance providers and about 35 per cent to private providers. (About 20 per cent of this last 35 per cent flows through private insurance funds and 80 per cent through out-of-pocket payments.) Theoretically the public sector covers over 70 per cent of the population, the social security sector over 20 per cent and the private sector about 2 per cent. However, this overstates the differences in coverage levels. In practice, as in other poor countries, the public sector achieves less than intended and public documents admit that about one-third of the population have no access to services while the private sector serves a much larger population who seek alternatives to both public- and social-insurance-provided services – about 20 per cent of the population. Although distributions vary between these three major sectors, this 'segmented' health system applies to all Latin American countries except Brazil, Chile, Argentina and Costa Rica. Colombia, most notably, is in the process of trying to reform from a 'segmented' to an integrated model.

Private, voluntary insurance plays an important role in a limited number of countries and always coexists with some form of coverage or compulsory arrangements for those it excludes, or would otherwise exclude. The USA is the most prominent country that substantially relies on this set of arrangements, with employers expected to provide coverage to their employees and dependants (61 per cent of the population are insured in this way), or individuals to insure themselves (13 per cent of the population). Public finance directly covers only the elderly, disabled and poor 23 per cent of the population. Arrangements for military veterans cover 4 per cent of the population. Fourteen per cent of the population are officially 'uninsured', although this group is indirectly able to access some services. The majority of providers are private, although there are some public health institutions that are established in areas the private sector fails to serve, such as inner cities. Until recently private insurance covered nearly 99 per cent of the population in Switzerland, although a share of the population was already covered compulsorily before this became universal in 1996. Significant subsidy also antedates the recent reforms. This extent of private, voluntary insurance is unequalled anywhere else in the world but some other countries also reach relatively high levels, including South Africa (where private insurance covers about 20 per cent of the population and accounts for about 50 per cent of expenditure) and Brazil, an otherwise 'integrated' exception to the 'segmented' Latin American model, but where 25 per cent of the population have private insurance.

These suggested categorisations are only points on the range of system options from the fully public to the fully private. Many health systems have different mixtures of the elements from the systems described above. Some have not been stable in their characteristics, even before the far-reaching and wide-ranging reforms of the 1990s. These have substantially changed the systems of many of the 'model' countries described above.

 Feedback

Often the facts about funding are rather different from the impression or beliefs people have. For example, the extent of co-payments is often overestimated because they are so visible compared with employer contributions to social insurance schemes.

Allocating public resources

The funding system should not channel public funds into low priority programmes and away from high priorities. The underlying reason is that spending on health care is inevitably limited (through the choices governments make to spend money on other areas such as private consumption, education and defence). Therefore decisions about which services to provide need to be made. This involves defining limits and setting priorities. The extent of health care that can be made available to all varies and in many low income countries this means providing access to only a basic set of essential services.

Priority setting is done through a process of distributing the inputs (usually funds) to health services, the *resource allocation process*. Resource allocation has two dimensions:

1 At the macro level, it is a planned process, based on policy decisions by government or public bodies, which devolves funds to purchasers (either central or local) or directly to providers.
2 At the micro level the amount of resources consumed by individual patients is determined by the professional judgement of health care workers.

There are three goals when allocating resources:

- *Equity*. You need to ensure that all people who need care have access to these services.
- *Allocative efficiency*. At both the macro and micro level it is necessary to ensure that funds are not wasted on services, which have, relative to other services, low effects on health.
- *Technical efficiency*. At the micro level, only the minimum necessary resources are used to deliver a particular activity or set of activities. Inefficiency may arise either if there is an inappropriate combination of inputs (e.g. health workers but no drugs or equipment) or an inappropriate use of inputs (e.g. using expensive hospital care when the same or better treatment could be provided at lower cost in primary care).

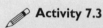 **Activity 7.3**

To integrate the various issues raised in this chapter, the following exercise will help you identify and discuss options for funding of health services and to appreciate that issues of financing health services are closely related to issues of health service provision.

The government of Fantasialand has engaged you to advise them on a new system of financing for their health services. They have decided to adopt a system of social insurance for the main funding, with some additional resources from co-payments (direct payment) and the state budget (taxation). However, many of the details of the new system are yet to be agreed and they have asked your advice on a series of questions. Fantasialand subscribes to the objectives of WHO Health for All, including the objective of ensuring affordable health services for the whole population.

Consider the following questions. None has a simple answer. For some there is an answer that is clearly wrong but normally the best answer depends on the objectives of the government.

1 Should there be one or more than one social insurance company?
2 Should the whole population be forced to subscribe to the scheme, or should richer people be allowed to make their own arrangements?
3 What should funds from taxes be used for? Should they be channelled through the insurance company or companies, used to pay for certain high cost services, such as haemodialysis and MRI scanning, or used as a direct subsidy to assist the participation of low income groups?
4 Should the premium be paid solely by the employee or should part of it be paid by the employer?
5 Membership of the insurance scheme will entitle people to health services. How should the level of entitlement be determined? What sort of services might be included or excluded?
6 Should people be free to choose any doctor and any hospital, with the costs paid by the insurance scheme?

↻ **Feedback**

1 The key concerns are the efficiency of risk bearing, choice and cost. Fewer companies will tend to allow more efficient spreading of risk, but there is less choice for the population. The effects on costs are not clear. If you believe that competition will lead to lower costs, then several should be allowed. If you believe that administration costs will be higher with many companies, then few should be allowed. There is also a problem of adverse selection (some companies avoiding taking on people who will need a lot of expensive care) if there are several companies.

2 Social insurance works on the principle of mutual support. Richer people contribute on average more than they take out, and poorer people less. If you allow richer people to opt out, then there is less mutual support, and the premiums for those who remain will be higher for any given level of service. This emphasizes that there are two purposes in collective funding – risk sharing and redistribution of resources. Allowing opt-outs does little to reduce risk sharing but reduces overall income.

3 It is tempting to believe that there is some advantage in certain high cost services being funded from taxation. But this is to confuse several arguments. Large insurance funds can share risk efficiently, so that there is no need to remove risk from them. The real danger of the state paying is that hard choices will not be made between routine and high cost care. The latter will be protected, whereas it might make more sense to spend less on high cost items and more on routine care. There is also the danger that the modest funds derived from taxation will be insufficient to maintain expensive but important specialist care. Another issue is how state funds can be used to subside those not in formal employment and with low incomes. For example, should subsidies be paid to the insurance company or companies to include them, or should subsidies be provided direct to health providers in order to give free care to this group?

4 The advantage of employee payment is that people are very conscious of the cost of health services. However, employers may be a powerful force to control health care costs.

5 The important point is that entitlements and contribution rates are connected, and the two decisions must be taken together.

6 This is a case of trade-off between administrative costs and choice. For free choice, all hospitals and all doctors need contracts with all insurance funds. Some countries have contracts with associations of hospitals or doctors, but this reduces the price competition. If capitation payment rather than fee-for-service is preferred, this inevitably limits choice to some degree.

Summary

The principal ways of funding include direct payments, private and social insurance and taxation. The overall objective of funding is to provide equitable and efficient health services. As health care resources are limited, funds should be directed to priority areas of care. Resources should be combined and distributed appropriately to improve health status at lowest cost.

You have now completed the section on inputs and will move on to learn about processes in the next four chapters.

References

McPake B, Kumaranayake L, Normand C (2002) *Health Economics – an International Perspective*. London: Routledge.

SECTION 3

Processes of health care

8 | The need and demand for health care

Overview

Now that you have looked at the inputs to care you will, following the systems approach of the book (Figure 1.1), move on to examine in more detail the processes (or activities) of health services.

The section starts with consideration of the concepts of need, demand and use. In this chapter you will explore the dimensions of need and the roles of illness behaviour and clinical judgement. In Chapter 9 you will look more closely at the various ways of measuring health services activity and at the sociodemographic factors influencing health services utilization. Chapter 10 invites you to explore the role of patients and gives an overview of the importance of staff–patient interaction. Finally, in Chapter 11 you will examine the ways in which lay people can influence health services policy either as individuals or collectively as members of communities.

Learning objectives

After working through this chapter, you will be better able to:

- understand the concepts of need, demand and use
- distinguish between different types of need
- outline the process of assessing the health care needs of populations.

Key terms

Clinical or professional judgement The decision taken by a clinician as to whether or not a patient has a normative need.

Demand Expressed need for health services.

Illness behaviour The way a person behaves when they feel a need for better health.

Relative need Comparison between needs of individuals with similar conditions or between needs of populations living in similar areas.

Use Utilization of health services that are actually provided.

A conceptual model of need, demand and use

The following model, which is represented diagrammatically in Figure 8.1, will help you to understand better the relationship between need and use.

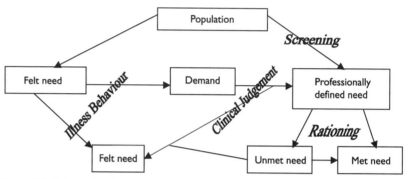

Figure 8.1 Relationships between need, demand and use

The process starts (at the top of the figure) with the population, some of whom have a subjective view that they have a *need for health* which, as you have seen in Chapter 4, is known as *felt need*. Depending on their personality, circumstances and beliefs, they may approach formal health services and make a *demand* (also referred to as *expressed need*). Alternatively, they may decide that the problem is not serious, will resolve without treatment or can be dealt with by lay care. Their felt need has not gone away but has not been turned into a demand for formal care. As you can see, people's *illness behaviour* will be a key determinant of the level of demand for formal care.

The next step is determined by the health care professional's reaction to the person's demand. *Clinical or professional judgement* determines whether or not the person's need for health is also a *need for health care*. If the clinician feels there is an appropriate (cost-effective) intervention available that the person could potentially benefit from, the clinician will confirm that a *normative need* exists. If not, the person will be discharged from formal care, albeit that they still have a need for health.

Those deemed to have a normative need will either be treated (*met need*) or they may have to wait until resources allow treatment (*unmet need*). This is known as *rationing*. Some normative need may never be met, if the necessary service does not exist, so they will remain with their felt need.

Returning to the population (at the top of the figure) there is one other circumstance to consider. There will be some people who feel fine and have no felt need but are harbouring the early stages of a disease (referred to as pre-symptomatic) or are at high risk of developing a disease. Most countries have some screening programmes to try and detect such people. Those found through screening will have a normative need but no felt need.

Activity 8.1

These concepts are illustrated by the following examples which describe four patients. Consider each and describe the situation using the terms you have learned above.

1 Patient A presents with abdominal pain. The surgeon diagnoses appendicitis and recommends an appendicectomy.
2 Patient B has osteoarthrosis of the hip and wants the joint to be replaced. The doctor approves of the demand and puts her on a waiting list.
3 Patient C has flu caused by a virus and demands drug treatment. There is no effective pharmaceutical intervention from which the patient could benefit.
4 Patient D is thought by his doctor to be suffering from depression and could benefit from treatment, but the patient is unconcerned.

Feedback

1 Clinical judgement approves of the demand for care. Felt need is congruent with normative need. The surgical intervention means their need is met.

2 Felt need and normative need are congruent but, due to rationing, need is not immediately met. It may be turned later into a met need.

3 There is no normative need. Clinical judgement has disapproved of the demand. The patient's felt need (for health) remains.

4 There is no felt need and so there is no expressed need. However, there is a normative need.

Need

As you have seen above and in Chapter 4, it is important to distinguish between different types of need. Recall that *felt need* depends on the judgement of the individual. It is subjective, determined by the individual's perceptions of their need for health. Measurement of the extent of felt need requires population surveys of self-assessed health.

Normative need depends on the judgement of professionals. Normative need varies over time and, as you have seen before, also with cultural context. The professional view is that to benefit from care there needs to be an effective intervention. An example of how normative need varies can be seen if you look at recommended policies for the use of routine cholesterol testing in different countries: in the USA it has been recommended for everyone over 20 years of age; in Canada for men aged 30–59 years; and in the UK it is not recommended (Savoie *et al.* 2000).

Differences in views of normative need affect whether or not whole services are provided. Comparing several European countries (including France, Switzerland, Germany, Netherlands), Polikowski and Santos-Eggimann (2002) found that while some services are included in publicly funded (taxation or social insurance) services everywhere (such as medical care, nursing home care, prescription drugs), other services are more controversial and not universally provided (such as dental care, home help, spas, chiropractic).

The third type of need is *unfelt need*. This depends on the existence of presymptomatic disease, which is not perceived by the individual.

In addition, there is the concept of *relative need*. This refers to the level of need of a population rather than a single individual. It is based on a simple comparison of the level of provision of a service in similar populations. If area A has more facilities than area B, the latter may be said to have a relative need. Such a judgement takes no account of whether or not the service in question is desirable (i.e. cost-effective) and should be provided anywhere.

Demand

Demand arises when need leads to action in search of care. So demand can be seen as *expressed* need. It depends on the following:

- *Felt need.*
- *Illness behaviour* – whether people take action to seek care depends on their perception of diseased status and cultural factors (see 'What is disease?' in Chapter 4).
- *Supply of services* – depends on two factors: the availability of facilities (buildings, staff, drugs, etc.) and the judgement of clinicians. The two are interrelated: if the number of beds in a hospital is doubled, the judgement of the clinicians may change such they now admit patients who previously were not admitted. In other words, the criteria that define normative need are altered.

Clinical judgement can also encourage or discourage demand for a service. For example, if a surgeon is not interested in a particular condition or operation, potential patients will be discouraged from seeking care. Similarly, a clinician with a special interest can attract additional patients (often referred to as *supplier-induced demand*).

Of course needs may *not* be expressed to formal carers. Unquestionably there are vulnerable groups who are less able to express their health care needs. But is there a large proportion of disease that doesn't receive formal care? This question was addressed by John Last, an Australian doctor, in the early 1960s. He concluded that there was a 'clinical iceberg', as illustrated in Figure 8.2. It suggests that the major proportion of need lies submerged below the surface and is not presented to formal carers.

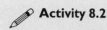 **Activity 8.2**

John Last concluded that some or all of the submerged iceberg should be hauled up above the surface so that more people received formal care. For each of the segments of the submerged iceberg, do you think such advice is well founded?

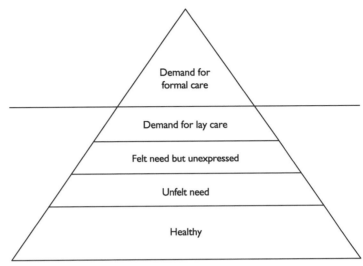

Figure 8.2 The clinical iceberg (based on Last 1963)

↻ **Feedback**

With the benefit of hindsight, Last's argument seems to be less convincing than when he made it in 1963. This is for several reasons, some of which you may have suggested:
1 'Demand for lay care' may be for conditions that do not require formal care such as many musculoskeletal conditions or minor psychological problems. Last's argument implies that people in this category would do better in the hands of formal carers than they are doing with lay carers. There is little evidence to support this.

2 Those with a 'felt need but unexpressed' may have made a considered decision to do nothing about their problem. To suggest such people ought to be demanding formal care is to encourage supplier-induced demand. It is an example of the innate tendency of formal carers to try and 'medicalize' people (as you saw in Chapter 3, sometimes referred to as medical imperialism).

3 Those with an unfelt need can only be detected by screening them. While many screening programmes have been demonstrated to be effective, many others remain controversial because the benefits to some people are outweighed by the harm and cost to others.

4 The 'healthy' should be encouraged to stay away from formal care!

Clinical judgement

As you have seen, whether demand for services is turned into use depends on the supply of services (availability and *clinical judgement*). Clinical judgement may vary between professionals. A simple example appeared in a British newspaper following a journalist visiting four dentists for a check-up (Collinson 1999). While one dentist's judgement was that nothing further needed to be done, the other three recommended dental care costing £96, £370 and a staggering £915!

You should be aware that variations in clinical decisions are common. Often it reflects an underlying lack of agreement as to what is the best form of treatment. However, it also may reflect other, less justifiable reasons. Professionals take decisions in the light of what is best for:

- *themselves* (aspiration for income; enjoyment of their work; desire for approval from their peers)
- *patients* (using every conceivable treatment regardless of cost)
- *third parties/society* (keeping to cost-containment policies of their employers and those paying for care; avoidance of their perceived risk of litigation).

All these are legitimate interests, which professionals need to keep in balance. Most health services problems are a result of a lack of balance between these three interests.

Needs assessment of populations

 Activity 8.3

Doctors routinely assess the needs of individual patients but how can they assess the health care needs of groups of patients? The article that follows on needs assessment by two public health doctors, Andrew Stevens and John Gabbay, examines some of the problems of *needs assessment of populations* and applies the needs, demand and use framework used in this chapter. While reading, focus on:

- the actors involved in needs assessment
- whose view should be considered to determine needs.

When you have finished reading, make fairly detailed notes in response to the following questions, drawing on what you have read.

1 Which professions and which organizations are involved in needs assessment in your country? Think, for example, of needs assessment for services for AIDS patients, the mentally ill, or mothers and children.
2 How would needs assessment based on felt need differ from one that focuses primarily on normative need? Think of potential conflicts between the views of professionals and of communities and the impact of both views on change of health services.

 Needs assessment, needs assessment . . .

A working definition of needs

Information about deprivation or mortality may tell us something about the need for health, but of itself says little about the need for health care. The two should not be confused. The need for health is related to the overall aim of a healthier population, but the need for health care is the current focus of needs assessment to improve the effectiveness of health services.

Therefore, in the present context, 'need' can be defined as the ability to benefit in some way from health care. After all, there can be no rational need for either an individual, or a population, to receive an item of care that confers no benefit. The ability of the population to benefit from health care depends on two things: the number of individuals affected, i.e. the incidence and prevalance of the condition under question, and the effectiveness of the services available to deal with it. Ideally, it will also take into account aetiological and other factors that are likely to influence the natural history of the disease or interfere with an intervention, but which are outside the scope of health services provision. Therefore, assessing needs must, at the very least, require us to have detailed information about those aspects of each condition for which we are considering the provision of preventive, diagnostic, therapeutic, rehabilitative and/or continuing care. Conditions will have to be defined quite clearly, and often sub-divided by severity, because each form of care may have only very narrow indications. Therefore despite the simple definition of needs there is a very large task, which is compounded by the interaction of need with demand and supply.

'Need', 'demand' and 'supply'

The distinction between need, demand and supply is well established, but further exploration is required in order to clarify the approach to 'needs' in service contracts, and to the information sources currently used for needs assessment.

. . . Need, demand and supply overlap. This means that there are eight potential fields – including the external field where a potential service is not needed, demanded or supplied (see Figure 8.3). A health care intervention for any specific condition will fit into one of these fields. Examples for the content of each field abound: in field 1, an example of what is needed, but neither supplied nor – on balance – demanded, might be a local proposal to increase substantially the rehabilitation facilities. Field 3 might include routine Caesarean sections on women with a history of a previous section, which is neither demanded nor needed but continues to be supplied. In field 5, an example of a service that is demanded and supplied, but not needed, would be the prescription of antibiotics for uncomplicated viral upper respiratory tract infection. Any useful assessment of needs will require not only an analysis of the relationship between need, demand and supply for the many conditions under consideration, but an attempt to see how the three can be made more congruent. Since all the fields are subject to change, the ideal would be to bring them closer together so that everything that is supplied is needed; and recognised as such by everyone. Health services would be more effective and also more efficient if as many services as possible were in field 7.

Information sources

The model (see Figure 8.4) may be used to demonstrate what information sources really tell us about needs in the context of supply and demand. The health service [in most or all countries] has always based its descriptions of need, however defined, on a variety of information sources. These include demographic data from the census, surveys on health status and on the views of patients, hospital utilisation rates, waiting lists, morbidity rates from registers and survey data, and (to a minor extent) studies on the effectiveness of interventions. Most of the routine sources are notoriously inaccurate, but even if they were perfect substantial problems would remain, not least because there are no generally agreed definitions of 'morbidity', or 'health problems', that will allow the unambiguous interpretation of the current diagnostic categories used in routine statistics.

Strictly, the assessment of needs, defined as the ability to benefit from care, would rely most heavily on detailed knowledge of morbidity rates and studies of effectiveness, which

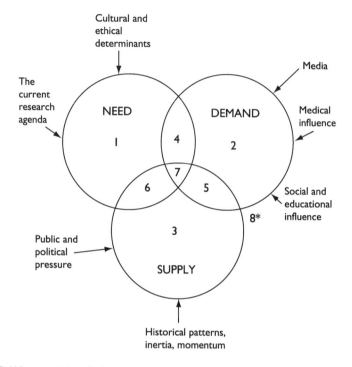

NEED: What people benefit from
DEMAND: What people ask for
SUPPLY: What is provided

* The external field where a potential service is
  not needed, demanded or supplied.

Figure 8.3 Need, demand and supply: influences and overlaps (Stevens and Gabbay 1991)

are relatively rare. However, since all the available routine information sources are being used in the current attempts at needs assessment, it is worth reviewing what they tell us. A few examples will suffice to highlight their limitations as measurements of need:

(i)   Waiting lists for surgery describe demand, which may be stimulated by supply, and which may or may not be needed (see Figure 8.4a).

(ii) Utilisation rates describe supply that may be either demanded, or needed, or both, or neither. Dental extractions, for example, may be performed for good clinical indications on people who prefer not to have them (a need not demanded), or at the patient's request when there is no clinical indication (a demand not needed), or even unscrupulously for profit (supplied, but neither demanded nor needed) (see Figure 8.4b).

(iii) Even morbidity information may tell a variety of stories. Cancer registry information does not in itself clarify the need for the treatment of, say, bronchial carcinoma, which can entail services that cover every combination of need, supply and demand (see Figure 8.4c). For example, where pneumonectomy does not alter a patient's prognosis, it is part of the supply that is not needed, but other forms of care, including preventive measures or continuing care, may confer benefit but be inadequately supplied, while

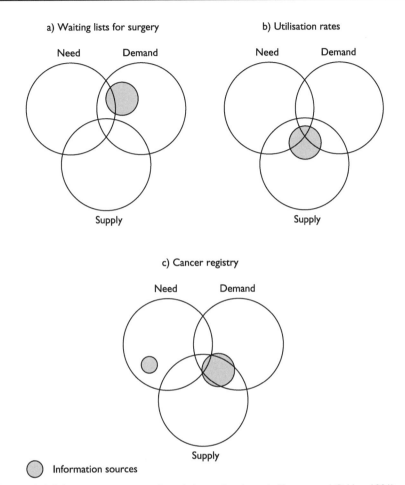

Figure 8.4 Information sources and need, demand and supply (Stevens and Gabbay 1991)

others will still be demanded whether needed or not. Hence morbidity data do not clarify the need for health care, unless complemented by a detailed knowledge of the effectiveness of services.

The current agenda

Clearly there are difficulties both with the meaning of need and with the value of the information available to assess it. Thus, although an epidemiologically sound assessment of needs is crucial to the development of health services, it will take a long time to produce.

. . . Firstly, there already exists a rough and ready epidemiological view of many needs, which should not be rejected on the grounds of its scientific impurity. For example, the shortcomings of the broad balance of care for ischaemic heart disease or child surveillance are already well enough known. A second standpoint . . . is to measure relative provision, which, without any other evidence, can provide clues to areas where changes are warranted. Thirdly, the preferences of local general practitioners are another powerful mechanism for improving the congruence between service contracts and local health needs . . .

The same can be said of consumer opinions, which are canvassed by many health author-ities as a step towards matching services to local demands, although often with the emphasis on the quality rather than the scale of services . . . Finally, there will always be managerial priorities dictated by central policy and modified by local considerations. The call for day surgery is a good example . . .

Conclusion

The very difficult task of assessing health needs will be aided by a clear distinction between need, supply and demand. This is important because successful adjustments to health care delivery will depend on how far need, supply and demand are made congruent. This success will in turn ultimately depend on a focused epidemiological research programme, but in the short term much can be done with the available tools.

 Feedback

Now compare your notes with the feedback below.

1 There are immense organizational and technical problems in assessing health care needs of the whole population. Most services are supplied without information on population need. Usually formal needs assessment focuses on defined health problems which are relevant to *changes in the provision of services*. Commonly, public bodies which commission or contract services have an interest in needs assessment. Ministries of health may have special planning units for this purpose or there may be joint commis-sions between government or social insurance corporations and the medical profes-sion. Ideally, needs assessment should be based on epidemiological data, which are applied to specific populations. If these are not available, assessing relative need may be the only feasible technique. Note that it is important to integrate professional views with the views of communities and other interest groups to increase accountability for the decisions.

2 Coordinating different professions and organizations as well as consumer views can be difficult. It may well be that the different actors don't take account of each other's view. Where clinical medicine is involved in needs assessment, it may be more influ-enced by patients' demand and the professional interests of doctors.

An approach based on felt need would incorporate the views of consumers and com-munities, whereas a normative needs approach is based on professional views. Focus on felt need could make services more responsive to consumers' needs. Emphasizing normative need is seen as less pertinent to change. For example, needs assessment may be used to justify existing services rather than to promote change.

Note that consumers and experts may have different priorities. As you will be aware by now, there is no neutral view of need. Several ways of reconciling community and professional views have been recognized (Hawe 1996):

a) The *functionalist* model of change as described above – this tries to synthesize data and views from different sources, including consumers' views, and gives managers the necessary information to shift resources.
b) The *conflict model of change* – this model focuses on consumers' demands and

builds on empowerment of communities to shift resources. Experts may participate in this process and address issues of normative need on behalf of the community but act within a consumer-defined framework.

Conflict-based strategies of needs assessment were successful in improving health services for deprived communities in the USA and Aboriginal health services in Australia. Think also of citizens opposing successfully the closure of a local hospital or groups demanding services for AIDS patients or for women's health needs.

 Activity 8.4

Before you finish this chapter, try answering the following questions, which will help you to revise the typology of social needs.

1 Fill in the terms.

The individually perceived variation from normal health is _____ need. Need that has led to action in search of formal care is called _____ . If a service one feels one needs is not available, need will not be _____ . Waiting lists can be used to measure _____ need. What experts define as need in a given situation is called _____ need. Comparison between health care provision of two similar populations allows an assessment of _____ need. Pre-symptomatic conditions are referred to as _____ need.

2 Which of the following statements is correct?

a) All felt needs should be treated by formal care.
b) Needs assessment of a population can be based on surveys of self-assessed health.
c) Assessment of relative need involves quantitative techniques to evaluate how local services differ from the norm.
d) Clinical judgement is sacrosanct and should not be questioned.

Feedback

Compare your answers with those below:

1 felt; demand; expressed; unmet; normative; relative; unfelt.

2 Statement (c) is the only correct one.

Summary

In this chapter you have read about the typology of health and health care needs. Felt need is determined by the individually perceived need for health. Depending on illness behaviour, felt need may be turned into an expressed need or demand for health care. Normative need depends on professional judgement. It is the capacity to benefit from care. Use of health services is strongly influenced by clinical judgement. Needs assessment is an important tool in deciding what services should be provided to meet health care needs at population level. While simple in principle, it is difficult in practice, which leaves policy makers dependent on using relative need to determine the services provided.

References

Collinson P (1999) Do dentists put the bite on patients? *The Guardian* 15 May.

Hawe P (1996) Needs assessment must become more change-focused. *Australian and New Zealand Journal of Public Health* 20: 473–8.

Last JL (1963) The iceberg: completing the clinical picture in general practice. *Lancet* ii: 28–31.

Polikowski M, Santos-Eggimann B (2002) How comprehensive are the basic packages of health services? An international comparison of six health insurance systems. *Journal of Health Services Research & Policy* 7: 133–42.

Savoie I, Kazanjian A, Bassett K (2000) Do clinical practice guidelines reflect research evidence? *Journal of Health Services Research & Policy* 5: 76–82.

Stevens A, Gabbay J (1991) Needs assessment needs assessment. . . . *Health Trends* 23: 20–3.

9 The relationship between need and use

Overview

In the previous chapter you explored the different types of need. In this chapter you will focus on the interrelationship between need and use. First, you will see how to measure use and how to analyse variations in utilization rates. Then you will explore the question of the extent to which use reflects need and, finally, learn about the inverse care law.

Learning objectives

After working through this chapter, you will be better able to:

- **give examples of ways of measuring use**
- **understand the causes of variations in utilization rates**
- **conceptualize the relationship between use and need.**

Key terms

Cross-boundary flow The use of services by people who are not resident in the local area of the facility.

Inverse care law The observation that availability of care appears to be inversely related to need.

Random variation Statistical differences that occur by chance and are inevitable when counting events.

Standardized mortality ratio (SMR) An indicator of the frequency of deaths in a population that takes into account the age and sex structure of the population.

Systematic variation Statistical differences that cannot be accounted for by the inevitable random variations that occur when counting events.

Utilization rate A measurement of health service use.

Measuring use of health services

In the previous chapter you learned about the factors that determine the use of health services. You will now explore how to measure use of health services and examine why utilization rates vary, internationally and within a country. The following activity asks you to reflect on the range of measurements of service use.

Utilization rates can either be *service-based* or *population-based*. Service-based rates use the number of people receiving care (such as the number of pregnant women cared for by community midwife) as the denominator. Population-based rates use the general population as the denominator.

Activity 9.1

Based on your experience, give examples from primary care and hospital care of some service-based and population-based rates.

Feedback

Your response will reflect your experience.

1 service-based rates (i.e. with no reference to the size of the population served):

- *primary care* – number of referrals to secondary care per primary care consultation; number of home visits per community nurse;
- *hospital care* – operations conducted as day care per 100 total (day care plus inpatient) operations.

2 Population-based rates:

- *primary care* – immunization coverage;
- *hospital care* – hospitalization rates.

Variation in utilization rates

Some examples will illustrate the extent to which variations in utilization exist around the world. Regardless of health care system, such variations are a universal feature.

Service-based rates

1 In the 1990s the number of referrals to hospital specialists made by general practitioners in Finland varied from 7 per 1000 consultations among the 20% of GPs with the lowest referral rates to 115 per 1000 amoung the 20% of GPs with the highest rates (Vehviläinen *et al.* 1996).

2 The proportion of operations to repair inguinal hernias (ruptures) performed as day cases in England in 1999/2000 varied between hospitals from less than 5% to over 80% (Figure 9.1).

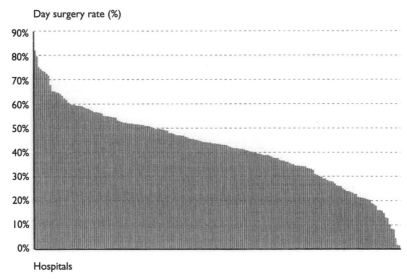

Figure 9.1 Variation in day surgery rates for inguinal hernia repair (England 1999/2000). There is still wide variation between hospitals (Audit Commission 2001)

Population-based rates

1 Measles immunization in 1997 varied (according to World Health Organization 1999) from 32% in Kenya to 100% in Iceland.
2 Hip replacement rates varied between districts of Ontario, Canada in 1995–97 from around 60 to 120 per 100,000 population, a two-fold variation (Badley and Williams 1998).
3 The proportion of babies born by Cesarean section varied from 1.4% to 16.0% among 18 Arab countries in the late 1990s. Rates were higher in countries in which the population was more urbanized, had higher literacy rates, higher gross domestic product, higher proportions of deliveries in hospitals, more physicians per capita, and lower fertility rates (Jurdi and Khawaja 2004).
4 The proportion of births attended by 'skilled health staff' in 1996–2000 varied from 10% in Ethiopia and 12% in Bangladesh, through 47% in Ivory Coast and 60% in Benin, to 88% in Brazil and 100% in Australia, according to the World Bank.

✎ **Activity 9.2**

Thinking back to Chapter 3, why might you be cautious in interpreting such data on birth attendants?

Feedback

> The implicit suggestion when using such a measure is that 'skilled health staff' are
> better than lay carers. While this may be true if there are difficulties with a delivery, for
> the vast majority of straightforward deliveries, a local lay person may be perfectly
> adequate.

What causes variation in use?

There are three categories of factors you need to consider when trying to explain
why variations occur.

1   Statistical factors:

    - *incomplete data* – you need to make sure information on all cases under con-
      sideration is included (e.g. private sector data may not be included);
    - *random variation* – observed differences may be due to chance.

2   Demand factors:

    - *age/sex composition* – varies between populations;
    - *morbidity rate* – frequency of the disease may vary;
    - *illness behaviour* – varies with cultural attitudes and sociodemographic
      characteristics.

3   Supply factors:

    - *availability of services* – number and distribution of facilities;
    - *professional judgement* – varies between clinicians.

Note that the main reason for *international variations* in utilization rates is the
availability of services. In addition morbidity rate, professional judgement and
illness behaviour have some influence. *Variations within a country* are likely to be
due to professional judgement and the availability of services.

 Activity 9.3

> Suppose the manager of a district hospital has observed that a certain operation is
> being performed more frequently than in the past and asks you to investigate possible
> causes. Having excluded the possibility of the increase being due to statistical factors,
> draw on what you have learned so far in this book to annotate the figure opposite with
> all the possible patient-related (demand) and health service-related (supply) factors
> that might influence:
>
> - the presentation rate to general practitioners
> - the referral rate to the district hospital
> - the intervention (surgical) rate.

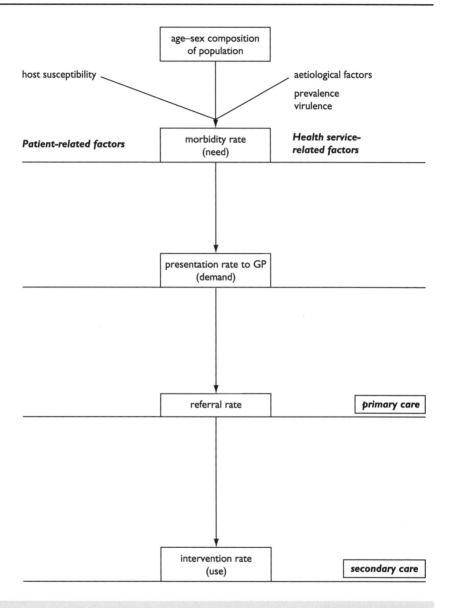

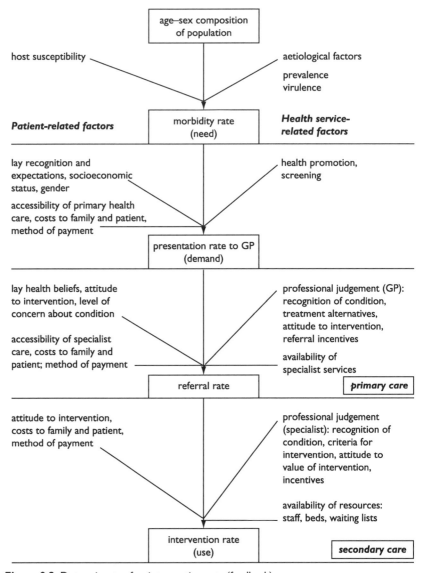

Figure 9.2 Determinants of an intervention rate (feedback)

Does use reflect need?

The finding that the use of health care varies between areas and over time is not, in itself, either a good or a bad thing. It may be that those who use more health care are sicker and, therefore, need more care. So does use reflect need? This is quite a difficult question to answer. It is known that use varies with at least two important social factors, age and socioeconomic status:

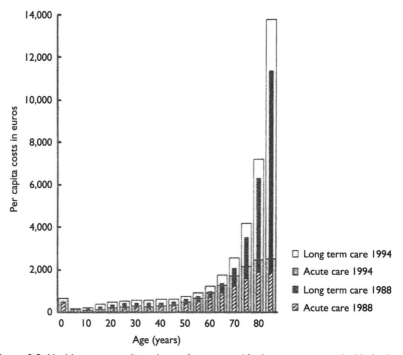

Figure 9.3 Health care expenditure by age for acute and for long term care in the Netherlands, 1994 and 1998 (Polder *et al.* 2002)

- *age* – health care is used more by elderly people and by infants. This can be seen in Figure 9.3, which shows how the level of health care expenditure varies with age in the Netherlands (Polder *et al.* 2002).
- *socioeconomic status* – health care is used more by less affluent people. This can be seen in all countries. In Catalonia, Spain, in 1994 this was observed both for ambulatory and hospital care (Borrell *et al.* 2001). Whereas 15% of men in the most affluent categories had visited a health care professional in the previous two weeks, 19.3% of the least affluent had. Similarly, the latter were more likely to have been hospitalized in the past year (8.8%) than the most affluent (6.1%).

A way of assessing the relationship between use and need is to calculate use–need ratios. One of the first attempts to do this was conducted in the UK in 1978 (Le Grand 1978). The level of need for each socioeconomic group was determined from a population survey of self-assessed health and the level of use was calculated using data from the health service. This showed that health care use for the most affluent socioeconomic group was 41% higher than for the least affluent group, having taken into account the greater level of need in the least affluent group.

Activity 9.4

Thinking about the types of need you learned about in Chapter 8, what do you think was the major limitation of such a comparison?

Feedback

The measure of need was that of felt need. Health services should be provided and used according to normative need that takes into account whether or not a cost-effective intervention exists.

Activity 9.5

A more recent attempt to compare use and need was carried out by Nick Black and colleagues. They looked at two surgical procedures that are common in high income countries, coronary artery bypass grafting and percutaneous transluminal coronary angioplasty used in treatment of coronary heart disease (CHD). Both methods are restricted to tertiary care centres and while most are carried out in the public hospitals (NHS), some take place in private hospitals. While reading the following edited version of the paper, don't worry about understanding the statistical analysis or technical details. The measure used to indicate variation in rates was the systematic component of variation. The larger the value, the greater the variation. Focus on the explanations for variations in use. Make notes on how the authors dealt with each of the possible explanations for variations in surgical rates: statistical, demand and supply factors.

Coronary revascularisation: why do rates vary geographically in the UK?

Wide variation has been reported in the utilisation rates of coronary artery bypass grafting (CABG) and percutaneous transluminal coronary angioplasty (PTCA) between regions of the United Kingdom, within North America, and between countries in Europe. The only factors to have been shown to be associated with the utilisation rate are the availability of facilities, in particular catheterisation laboratories, and the distance patients live from these facilities. No association has been found with the rate of use of alternative therapies and the level of coronary heart disease morbidity in the population.

In an attempt to understand the reasons for variation in revascularisation rates in the UK . . . this paper describes analyses of the variations that occurred during 1992–93 [in four regions of the country].

Results

Amount of variation in NHS crude rates

Rates of CABG varied between districts almost fivefold from 226 to 1015 per million population aged 25 years or more (Figure 9.4). PTCA rates varied much more, from 12 to 1450 per million. The greater degree of variation for PTCA was seen by comparing the systematic component of variation (SCV) for the two procedures for each region (Table 9.1). Apart from in Greater Glasgow (which comprised only three districts) the SCV for PTCA was much higher than that for CABG.

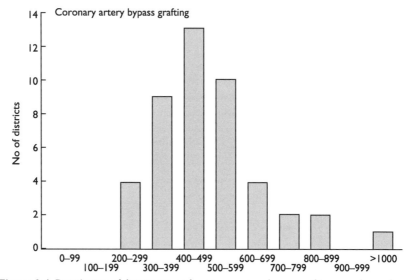

Figure 9.4 Distribution of district rates of coronary artery bypass grafting – crude number of NHS cases per million population aged 25 years and over, 1992–93 (Black *et al.* 1995)

Statistical reasons

The first possible explanation considered was that data might have been missing for those districts with the lowest rates as a result of incomplete data collection in the hospitals, incorrect clinical coding, or failure to allow for cross-boundary flows. However, the data were collected directly from clinical departments rather than relying on hospital information systems, so we are confident that few if any cases were missed and that the coding of operative procedures was accurate . . .

Demand factors

The demand for any procedure depends on three factors: the normative need for treatment, people's expectations, and the use of alternative interventions. The normative need is determined partly by the age–sex structure of the population and the prevalence of coronary heart disease in the population. Direct standardisation for age and sex had no impact on the degree of variation. Indeed, the SCVs for age–sex standardised rates were larger than those for the crude rates (Table 9.1).

Table 9.1 Extent of inter-district variation of crude and age–sex standardized revascularisation rates within each region measured by the systematic component of variation. NHS and private cases included except in south east Thames region (NHS only)

	Health region			
	E Anglian	N Western	SE Thames	G Glasgow
Coronary artery bypass grafting				
NHS crude rates	4.6	12.1	5.7	6.6
NHS + private crude rates	5.6	9.4	[5.7]	8.1
NHS + private standardised rates	9.8	12.0	12.5	8.1
Percutaneous transluminal coronary angioplasty				
NHS crude rates	14.8	59.9	50.4	2.9
NHS + private crude rates	21.8	41.0	[50.4]	3.4
NHS + private standardised rates	23.7	44.7	60.1	4.1

Source: Black *et al.* (1995).

As no accurate epidemiological data on disease prevalence exist, proxy measures were used: the standardised mortality ratio for coronary heart disease and two measures of social deprivation (which has been shown to be related to the prevalence of coronary heart disease). Age–sex standardised revascularisation rates were inversely correlated with SMRs but were positively correlated with social deprivation (Figure 9.5) . . . In other words, higher intervention rates were associated with districts with lower SMRs and with more deprived districts.

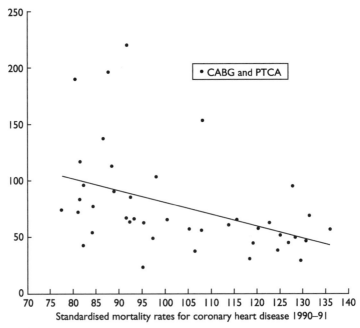

Figure 9.5 Relationship between district utilisation rates for revascularisation (1992–93) with standardised mortality ratios for coronary heart disease (1990–91) (Black *et al.* 1995)

Demand for either CABG or PTCA could be affected by the use of the other procedure. In practice, the opposite occurred. The regional age–sex standardised rates (NHS plus private) for CABG were highly correlated with those for PTCA (Pearson correlation coefficient $r = 0.81$; 95% confidence interval (0.63, 0.90)).

Supply factors

It was not possible to relate district utilisation rates to the availability of tertiary or specialist services as services are not specifically allocated to each district. It was possible, however, to relate regional rates to the availability of regional services. This showed that both CABG and PTCA rates correlated with consultant and non-consultant staffing levels but not with bed numbers. Generally the higher the staffing level, the higher the utilisation rate . . .

Two indicators of service availability at district level were used. Firstly, the influence of the distance of the district from the main specialist centre was investigated by mapping. This showed that, in general, the closer a district was to a centre the higher was the rate. The second indicator used was whether or not a district had a local cardiologist . . . Of the seven districts which did not have a cardiologist, the mean rate for CABG was 378 per million, compared with 535 per million for the other 38 districts ($p = 0.041$). The equivalent rates for PTCA were 89 and 306 per million ($p = 0.007$).

Discussion

Rates of coronary revascularisation vary geographically within the UK principally because of differences in the supply of services. This study has shown that significant differences in regional and district rates persist even when statistical and demand factors have been taken into account. These geographical differences can partly be explained by differences in the availability of specialist revascularisation services, such as levels of medical staffing in regional centres, the presence of a local cardiologist and the distance from a specialist centre. As such our results are consistent with previous findings.

Any remaining differences may be due to variation in clinical judgment about the appropriate indications for intervention. As a standard method for recording patients' clinical indications for treatment is not employed routinely in the UK, it was not possible in this study to investigate how clinical judgment varied between the specialist centres . . .

 Feedback

Your completed table should show much of the following information:

Statistical factors. Data completeness was ensured by direct data collection from clinical departments, rather than using hospital information systems. Both public and private providers (hospitals) were included. Random variation was taken into account by using standard statistical probability tests that give an indication of whether or not a difference between districts was due to chance.

Demand factors. Age–sex composition of the population was taken into account by adjusting the data in the comparisons (using standardization). Morbidity rate was measured using the standardized mortality ratios for CHD as a proxy measure; this approach may be inaccurate but often direct measures of disease prevalence are not available. Socioeconomic status was taken into account using a social deprivation index based on census data.

Supply factors. Availability of services was obtained from local staff. The distance of each district from a tertiary centre was obtained from maps. The findings were similar to those of Le Grand thirty years earlier: use of surgery was higher in districts with lower levels of need. Recently, the same relationship between socioeconomic status and use of coronary surgery was observed in Rome, Italy (Ancona *et al.* 2000). They found that the most affluent men had surgery at the rate of 14.1 per 100 cases of CHD compared to only 8.9 per 100 among the least affluent. These findings are consistent with an observation made several decades ago and known as the inverse care law.

The inverse care law

By now you have seen many examples which demonstrate that use does not reflect need. Moreover, service availability often appears to be inversely related to need. This relationship was described by Julian Tudor Hart, a GP working in Wales, in 1971:

> In areas with most sickness and death, general practitioners have more work, larger lists, less hospital support, and inherit more clinically ineffective traditions of consultations than in the healthiest area; and hospital doctors shoulder heavier case loads with less staff and equipment, more obsolete buildings and suffer recurrent crises in the availability of beds and replacement staff. These trends can be summed up as the inverse care law: that availability of good medical care tends to vary inversely with the need of the population served.

Summary

Use can be assessed by service-based and population-based measurements. Utilization rates vary internationally and within a country, depending on several demand and supply factors. The key question is whether use of services reflects health care needs. Analysis must take account of the sociodemographic factors affecting need and consider use–need ratios to analyse whether higher utilization rates reflect higher levels of need. Socioeconomic status is an important determinant not only of morbidity and mortality but also of health care utilization. This fact requires careful consideration when planning and evaluating health services.

References

Ancona C, Agabiti N, Forastiere F *et al.* (2000) Coronary artery bypass graft surgery: socio-economic inequalities in access and in 30 day mortality. A population-based study in Rome, Italy. *Journal of Epidemiology & Community Health* 54: 930–5.

Audit Commission (2001) *Acute Hospital Portfolio. Review of National Findings. Day Surgery.* London: Audit Commission for England and Wales.

Badley EM, Williams JI (1998) *Patterns of Health Care in Ontario: Arthritis and Related Conditions.* Toronto: Institute for Clinical Evaluative Sciences.

Black NA, Langham S, Petticrew M (1995) Coronary revascularisation: why do rates vary geographically in the UK? *Journal of Epidemiology & Community Health* 49: 408–12.

Borrell C, Fernández E, Schiaffino A, Benach J, Rajmil L, Villalbí JR, Segura A (2001) Social class inequalities in the use of and access to health services in Catalonia, Spain: what is the influence of supplemental private health insurance? *International Journal of Quality in Health Care* 13: 117–25.

Hart JT (1971) The inverse care law. *Lancet* i: 405–12.

Jurdi R, Khawaja M (2004) Caesarean section rates in the Arab region: a cross-national study. *Health Policy & Planning* 19: 101–10.

Le Grand J (1978) The distribution of public expenditure and the case of health care. *Economica* 45: 125–42.

Polder JJ, Bonneaux L, Meeding WJ, van der Maas PJ (2002) Age-specific increases in health care costs. *European Journal of Public Health* 12: 57–62.

Vehviläinen AT, Kumpusalo EA, Voutilainen SO, Takala JK (1996) Does the doctors' professional experience reduce referral rates? Evidence from the Finnish referral study. *Scandinavian Journal of Primary Health Care* 14: 13–20.

World Health Organization (1999) *The World Health Report. Making a Difference.* Geneva: WHO.

Staff–patient interactions

Overview

In this and the next chapter you will look at the users of health systems and examine their roles as patients and members of the public. In this chapter the focus of analysis is on users in the role of patients. You will explore the problems of staff–patient interaction in health services and the psychosocial factors affecting the process of communication.

Learning objectives

After working through this chapter, you will be better able to:

- **outline factors that influence the style of staff–patient interaction**
- **suggest reasons for failure to communicate with patients**
- **give examples of how to improve the staff–patient relationship.**

Key terms

Bureaucracy A formal type of organization involving hierarchy, impersonality, continuity and expertise.

Compliance The extent to which a patient follows professional advice.

Empathy A response that demonstrates understanding and acceptance of the patient's feelings and concerns.

Encounter The interaction of two or more people in a face-to-face meeting.

Social role A set of ideas and actions that let individuals behave according to expected social norms.

Lay people as patients, consumers and communities

In Chapter 6 you explored power as a key concept in understanding professionalism and identified the attributes of professional power. One aspect of this and the following chapter is an exploration of the relative power of lay people. Note that different terms for lay people are used:

- *Patients* are people expressing a felt need for better health in an *interpersonal* relationship with health workers.

- *Consumers* are lay people who are aware of their knowledge, making choices and influencing the distribution and use of power. Think of informed people selecting providers and insurance companies in competitive health care markets (Chapter 7). In the consumerist view, people are seen as *customers* of health services.
- *Communities* may be regarded as the 'public' participating in health care issues – self-defined groups sharing something in common and recognizing a collective experience (e.g. local residents, the Hispanic community). Remember the different forms of interaction with communities in needs assessment and how the functionalist and the conflict model relate to different levels of empowerment.

Most of the research in high income countries has focused on the interaction between staff and patients. The primary focus of this chapter is on staff. The next chapter will look more closely at the role of people as consumers and as members of communities.

Why study staff–patient interaction?

There are many reasons for practitioners and managers to be aware of the importance of staff–patient interaction. Poor communication between staff and patients is a major reason for dissatisfaction and poor outcome of care.

One study in the UK in the early 1990s found the commonest criticisms of general practitioners were: inadequate clinical treatment (27%), practitioner not responding or cooperating (27%), personal attributes of health professional (25%), organization of practice/staff (10%), financial issues (7%) and mistakes by practitioner (4%). The authors concluded that the doctor's 'ability to dispense pills is not in question but his manner – abrupt and abrasive – calls into question his ability as a general practitioner' (Nettleton and Harding 1994). This was consistent with a previous study which reported patients' views of the relative importance of different attributes. Most important was that the doctor provided sufficient information, next that the doctor was 'likeable', then that the consultation was long enough and only fourth in importance, that the doctor had good medical skills (Williams and Calnan 1991).

The impact of communication between staff and patients on outcomes of care is well documented. For example, instruction and encouragement of patients can reduce post-operative pain (Egbert 1964). Patients who received extra visits from anaesthetists were able to leave hospital three days earlier.

In the USA, studies into the high frequency of litigation suggest that failure to communicate adequately with patients is a main reason (Levinson *et al.* 1997). Failure to communicate with patients is related to three areas:

- *Failure to assess the full spectrum of patient concerns*. In a study of routine encounters, patients were typically interrupted after 18 seconds.
- *Failure to develop and maintain therapeutic relations* – empathy, a response demonstrating an accurate understanding and acceptance of a patient's feelings. Developing empathy reduces negative emotions such as anger, anxiety and depression, which are common reactions to illness.
- *Failure in delivering information to patients*. Levels of distress are reduced when

patients perceive themselves to have received adequate information on diagnostic procedures and treatment plans. Most challenging for staff is communicating bad news to patients and their families.

Activity 10.1

Poor interaction leading to patient dissatisfaction is not restricted to affluent people in high income countries. The following article by Michael Bernhart and colleagues (1999) describes a study carried out in Indonesia in 1998 which tried to overcome people's reluctance to criticize health services. As you read it consider:

1   How did the researchers try and achieve this?
2   How successful were they?
3   What were the principal sources of dissatisfaction?

 ### Patient satisfaction in developing countries

There have been several efforts to elicit constructive criticism from clients of Indonesian health care facilities, but the responses from clients have been uniformly laudatory. As examples: a survey of 4000 patients of a primary care facility in Jakarta found that 94.7% of the respondents were fully satisfied. A similar survey of 1200 patients in three health centers conducted by the East Java Province Health Office found the satisfaction rate at 93.2% . . . They are almost certainly not representative of true feelings given that drop-out rates from preventive and chronic curative services range from 25 to 35% and less than one in four citizens uses the public sector primary care facilities. More intensive grilling of patients does not seem to change the result; a similar finding was produced in a study of women in West Java using antenatal care services which solicited opinions on 12 areas of client satisfaction (Sinyor, 1997). The interviewing was intensive (average duration of interview was 78 min); yet no respondent answered that she was dissatisfied with a single aspect of the services (5.3% did voice only moderate satisfaction with a few items). Again, the drop-out rate belies the rosy image projected by the results.

Research questions

If Indonesian patients normally withhold negative opinions or evaluative comments, would they be more forthcoming with factual information, even though that too might be interpreted negatively? The study reported in this paper addresses that question. The practical relevance of the question is that useful information on patient satisfaction might be obtained if clients are asked about events and behaviors, rather than for their opinions.

. . . A second challenge, not specific to Indonesia, is to identify those aspects of the service that are meaningful to patient satisfaction. Although a number of patient satisfaction studies have been conducted in Indonesia, it does not appear that any of them methodically determined the relevance to patients of the variables employed . . .

Method

A list of 14 factors thought to be potentially relevant to patient satisfaction was compiled. These factors came from examination of literature reviews on patient satisfaction and a series of focus groups conducted by Rusmiyati (1997) in West Java. These factors were framed in terms of events and observable behaviors, not opinions. To illustrate, patients were not asked whether they felt acceptable norms of privacy were observed, but rather they were asked whether anyone was present during examination, counselling and treatment who did not participate in providing care ... Two of the 25 questions did elicit opinions: facility cleanliness, where the researchers could not agree on an objective indicator; and speed of service. The latter was to check perceptions of the wait against actual recorded time spent in the clinic.

Seventy-five patients were interviewed in 11 clinics on three islands. The islands were chosen to sample the breadth of diversity of Indonesia ...

Results

Table 10.1 summarizes the findings on relative importance and the frequency of expressed negative information.

Table 10.1 Relative importance of patient satisfaction factors and frequency of negative responses

Patient satisfaction area	Importance score	Negative responses
To be cured	0.89	23%
Receive medicine	0.78	4
Privacy during examination	0.58	28
Cleanliness of the facility	0.57	65
Receiving full information on the name, nature, prognosis, management, and danger signs	0.55	38
Receiving intelligible answers to questions	0.53	20
Receiving encouragement to ask questions	0.52	75
Use of the household/indigenous language	0.44	11
Continuity of provider	0.41	51
Waiting time for service and total wait	0.40	14, 31 min
Availability of a toilet	0.33	0
Cost of the service	0.31	1
Availability of a seat	0.30	1
Health worker engaging patient in social conversation	0.27	73

Source: Bernhart et al. (1999).

Frequency of critical or negative information

It may be observed from the right-hand column that negative responses were forthcoming from patients in far greater percentages than had been obtained in earlier opinion-based research. As examples of the constructive criticism offered, 28% of the respondents answered that someone not participating in their health care service had been present during the examination, 38% had not received information and 65% faulted the cleanliness of the facility ...

Relative importance

The center column reports the relative ratings of importance; the range is from 0 (least important) to 1.0 (most important). With rare exceptions (eight of the 75 respondents) patients ranked being cured as the most important aspect of the service. This was hardly unexpected, but its first place finish provided reassurance that the answers on relative importance were not given without thought. Patients ranked receiving medicine as second most important and privacy as the third. There were further questions regarding privacy for women who were required to disrobe for the examination. Against expectations, privacy was nearly as important an aspect of care for men as for women.

As may be seen in Table 10.1, the top ranked issues were associated with medical aspects of care (cure and medicine), followed, loosely, by issues concerning personal dignity and completeness and intelligibility of counseling. Surprisingly, 'obvious' satisfaction issues such as cost, continuity, waiting time and amenities were relegated to the bottom of the list. However, the low cost of service, built-in continuity of provider in the smaller facilities and widespread availability of amenities may have diminished patient concern with these factors.

Consistency of responses among respondents

As noted earlier, given the heterogeneity of the society, there was concern that respondents of different cultural backgrounds would assign different relative importance to the factors. It appears that they did not. The consistency of response was assessed across regions, sexes and purpose of visit to the facility; only the last produced variation.

There was no statistically detectable difference among relative rankings of importance by region . . .

Discussion

. . . The assertion that patients were willing to provide critical information should, perhaps, be rephrased to read that they will provide more critical information. Although the politeness bias seems to give way when factual information, not opinions, are requested, we cannot determine whether the responses are fully candid. It was possible, however, to test the plausibility of some of the answers given. The five questions on counseling were all followed by a request to the patient to describe the information given; their answers were recorded and later rated for plausibility by an individual who did not collect the data. This is a slippery concept, to be sure, but the research was not concerned with the accuracy of the counseling given – simply whether counseling was provided as claimed by the patient – and the patients' answers were scored as 'plausible' if the content of their answer was something a health worker could have plausibly said.

 Feedback

1 People were asked about events and behaviours, rather than for their opinions. It was hoped that if patients asked for information that might be verified, they would be more likely to answer based on their experience in the clinic.

2 Negative responses were forthcoming from patients in far greater percentages than had been obtained in earlier opinion-based research.

3 Not encouraged to ask questions (75%); health worker did not engage patient in social conversation (73%); facility not clean (65%); and lack of continuity of provider (51%).

Compliance and staff–patient interaction

Compliance has been defined as the extent to which patients follow professional advice. Though socioeconomic and cultural factors play an important role, staff–patient interaction also influences compliance with treatment (Sbaro and Sbaro 1994). Take, for example, tuberculosis control. Though short term combination chemotherapy is effective and inexpensive, TB is still the major infectious cause of death worldwide. Notwithstanding the logistical difficulties of case detection in low income countries, failure of compliance with treatment is considered a global problem. High proportions of patients discontinue medication when they feel better but stay infectious and communicate the disease. Hopes are directed towards the development of even shorter treatment regimes, but effective interaction of health workers with patients forms a central part of any control strategy. As an example from Bangladesh demonstrates, specially trained village health workers who are trusted by local communities achieve high rates of case detection and treatment compliance (Chowdhury *et al.* 1997).

Factors influencing the staff–patient encounter

A variety of factors influence staff–patient encounters. Among these are:

- patient's socioeconomic status
- severity of disease
- the type of setting (home care/institutional care)
- patient's knowledge
- the method of paying for care.

 Activity 10.2

The following extracts – mostly from the UK and drawn from an Open University book (U205 Course Team 1985) – give an introduction to problems arising from poor staff–patient communication. As you read them, consider the following:

1 For each encounter, whether it was considered satisfactory by the patient and by the doctor/nurse. If not, why not?
2 The conversational style of, on the one hand, the doctors and the nurses and, on the other hand, the patients.
3 The impact, if any, that the method of payment had on the encounters.

 Analysing staff–patient encounters

1 A consultation between a male GP and a female patient taken from a study of 71 GPs who, with their patients' permission, tape recorded their consultations – around 2500 in all (Byrne and Long 1976):

DOCTOR Come in, please, come in and sit down. No better?
PATIENT I don't know what was the matter, but I've had a fortnight in bed.
DOCTOR With what?

PATIENT With flu.

DOCTOR Flu?

PATIENT I lost my balance.

DOCTOR And how did this flu affect you?

PATIENT I was sweating and sneezing, I couldn't stop sneezing.

DOCTOR Any aches and pains?

PATIENT Well, I was all aching, all over.

DOCTOR Any cough?

PATIENT Yes, I had a cough.

DOCTOR Bad?

PATIENT Well, it was really like bronchitis. I got a lot up, it was that greeny colour.

DOCTOR No blood?

PATIENT Oh, no.

DOCTOR Has that cleared now? The phlegm.

PATIENT Well, no, not quite, it's still loose on the chest.

DOCTOR You still get it up? Still green?

PATIENT Yes.

DOCTOR . . . [indistinct]

PATIENT Rusty again.

DOCTOR Are you taking those tablets I gave you?

PATIENT Oh, yes, I'm still taking those tablets.

DOCTOR Have you got any pain in your chest?

PATIENT No. There's no more pain.

DOCTOR Are you short of breath?

PATIENT Oh, yes, I get that. You see, when I was short of breath before, I used to get the pain.

DOCTOR Gone completely, has it?

PATIENT Yes.

DOCTOR That's something.

PATIENT But during the night, sometimes, I can feel it like catarrh at the back of my throat. But that looks brown.

DOCTOR Does it wake you? Your chest.

PATIENT Well, it's not these last few nights.

DOCTOR These little white tablets, have you any left?

PATIENT No . . .

DOCTOR What's your weight doing now, steady?

PATIENT Well, as a matter of fact, Doctor, we were weighing ourselves last night, my husband and I, and he said, 'What weight are you?' and I said, 'According to those I'm only eight stone', and we put it past the zero and it was only eight stone odd.

DOCTOR . . . [indistinct]

PATIENT So I don't think . . . [indistinct] the scale for a while. I think I was eight stone two when you weighed me last.

DOCTOR You were eight stone four, you have lost a bit.

PATIENT Yes, I have.

DOCTOR That's reasonable, because the thyroid tablets . . . I'll make a note of that. Well, keep on the white tablets, one a day. I'll give you some tablets and medicine to clear your chest, the instructions will be on the bottle.

PATIENT . . . everyone has a cold.

DOCTOR It's a bad time of year; you take the tablets four times a day and the medicine according to the instructions, I think you'll find that will clear it. There is enough there anyway for about a week. If you are not 100 per cent certain, you must come back. But the little white tablets you must take permanently. So see how you get on and if you're not happy come back in a week.

PATIENT I see Andrew's had a bad cold, hasn't he?

DOCTOR Has he?

PATIENT He's still sniffly.

DOCTOR Well, it's the time of year for it, you can't expect . . .

PATIENT . . . but I could have done with trying those flu injections . . .

DOCTOR It's too late this year now.

PATIENT Yes, it's too late.

DOCTOR About November.

PATIENT I'll come in then.

DOCTOR Well, last year was a good year for flu and this year isn't so good.

PATIENT My throat is a bit . . .

DOCTOR When you get an infection you will always get this rustiness . . .

PATIENT I noticed that . . . Dr X told me I had a relaxed throat. I had to not speak as much and stop singing so I can't get the high notes now. All my notes have gone.

DOCTOR Bye now.

2 Some short extracts recorded by another researcher, this time a nurse, Jill Clark (1981). She asked nurses (all female) on surgical wards to wear a small microphone dipped to their uniform. The extracts below illustrate what she found.

NURSE How are you feeling this morning?

PATIENT A Hungry.

NURSE Ah well, I'm afraid there's nothing we can do about that, just at the moment.

PATIENT A But . . .

NURSE You can have any fluids you like – but just stick on the fluid diet at the moment.

NURSE There we are dear, OK? [gives tablet]

PATIENT B Thank you. Do you know, I can't feel anything with my fingers nowadays at all.

NURSE Can't you?

PATIENT B No, I go to pick up a knife and take my hand away and it's not there anymore.

NURSE Oh, broke my pen! [moves away]

NURSE Did they find you an interesting case?

PATIENT C They did, yes.

NURSE That's nice. Can I just rub your bottom then?

PATIENT C But they um . . .

NURSE One, two, three . . . up. Not getting sore, sitting here, are you?

PATIENT C Well I am a little bit sore.

NURSE Are you walking around a little bit with your [colostomy] bag so you don't get too sore?

3 Unfortunately, there has been very little research into the characteristics of private practice. Two small studies of private medical consultation do exist, however. The first excerpt is from a private paediatric clinics in the USA (Strong 1979), the second from a private oncology (cancer) clinic in London (Silverman 1984).

INTERN [a junior doctor who sees the patient before the specialist] How did you get here?

MOTHER Well, he's been seeing a psychiatrist and he diagnosed minimal brain dysfunction and prescribed X. But we also want to get Dr Stein's [a neurologist] opinion as we felt we ought not just to have a psychiatric opinion.

MR J I'm a member of PPP [a private insurance scheme] and so if you send them the account they will pay . . . They asked for a report if you can send one.

DOCTOR What shall I say?

MR J Whatever you think.

DOCTOR No, what you say. I'm your agent. I'll write whatever you want.

Feedback

1 You are likely to have used words such as helpless or frustrated when describing the feelings of the patients in the first four encounters. At the same time, the doctors or nurses in these encounters did not seem to find them satisfying either.

2 The doctor asks a lot of quick-fire questions, 17 in all, which produce short, snappy answers. He moves rapidly from one topic to another as do the nurses, who also have a quick-fire style composed of questions, comments and instructions. Both the doctor and two of the nurses interrupt remarks by patients and you may also have noticed that in two of the extracts staff end the interaction while patients are still trying to talk. Indeed, neither the doctor nor the nurses respond in a particularly inviting way to patients' comments and questions.

In contrast to the very precise manner of staff, patients have a far more conversational, even rambling style on occasions, in which some things are described in an anecdotal, story-telling fashion – for example, 'Well, as a matter of fact, Doctor, we were weighing ourselves last night, my husband and I, and he said . . .'. Note also that the patient consulting the doctor does not ask nearly so many questions, nor, like the other patients, does she object when her remarks are overridden. Finally, you may have noticed that relatively little technical information is passed on from staff to patient.

3 The balance of power changed when patients were paying for their treatment. The doctors appeared to listen more and to 'dictate' less to the patients. The patients appeared to feel more 'in control'. Generally, the form of payment can be a strong incentive to change behaviour in interaction with patients. Depending on the setting, one might also note that private patients get a friendlier encounter but not necessarily better care. You may also find that private (or non-governmental) facilities have a different management style, with more opportunities for staff development than in government facilities, affecting their behaviour towards patients. Choice of doctors in primary and secondary care may also increase regard for consumer concerns.

The following activity invites you to reflect on the importance of interpersonal skills for health services performance.

Activity 10.3

1 How can staff communicate better with patients?
2 If you have worked as a clinician, reflect on your own experience – have you had systematic training in interpersonal skills?

 Feedback

1 From what you have read, you may have concluded that staff with good interpersonal skills will contribute most to patient satisfaction. The teaching of these important skills is increasingly included in professional education of health care workers.

2 It is important to be aware that interpersonal skills can be systematically taught: there are examples of communication training being successfully integrated into education of primary health care workers and family planning staff in low income countries.

Societal forces shaping the staff–patient encounter

You have looked at the different styles of the staff–patient encounter. But what are the forces underlying this relationship? What makes patients and staff act as they do? Sociological research has identified some general principles underlying the staff–patient interaction. Cross-cultural research suggests that these can be found in all cultures. Relative power and routine work are important concepts explaining the position of patients.

- *Relative power*. Patients are in a weak bargaining position. They are vulnerable and helpless, and many are ill informed about their status. The experience of illness leads them to seek a passive role. However, this situation is changing in high income countries as patients gain confidence and acquire knowledge about their condition (see below).
- *Routine work*. Patients are treated as objects of work and each client is one of many. What a patient perceives as a unique situation is routine for the staff.

Two influences on the staff–patient relationship are *cultural norms* and *bureaucracy*.

Cultural norms

Talcott Parsons was one of the earliest sociologists to investigate the relationship between doctors and patients. Both doctors and patients are regarded as occupying *social roles*, which facilitate their interaction and define the expected behaviour of each.

Parsons is associated with the *functionalist* perspective (Parsons and Mayhew 1982). Society is seen as a system in which each element serves a purpose or maintains a function; members of society fulfil their *roles* to meet society's needs because they share common goals and values. The role an individual occupies is related to social status and represents a set of ideas and actions. Social functioning is achieved by individuals acting according to their expected role. For example, the *sick role* ensures social functioning by expecting people to behave according to social norms: unlike other forms of absenteeism, sick leave is socially accepted. But employees are expected to return to work as soon as possible, as sick leave rates that are too high would impair economic performance.

Remember also from previous chapters the functionalist view on women's role in lay care and on the role of doctors as professionals. Though the functionalist perspective was influential in the 1950s, it has been criticized for taking too little account of change and conflict in society.

In Parsons' view, both roles, the patient's (the 'sick' role) and the doctor's, involve privileges and obligations. *Privileges* of the sick role include:

- the right to be exempted from normal activity (e.g. not going to work)
- being regarded as in need of care and not being blamed for one's illness.

Obligations involve:

- to seek medical advice
- to want to get well as quickly as possible.

In turn, doctors are granted the *privileges*:

- to examine patients physically and psychologically
- of professional autonomy and authority.

Doctors have the *obligations*:

- to be objective and neutral (e.g. not to judge patients' behaviour on moral grounds)
- to use professional skills for the welfare of patients and the community (rather than for self-interest).

Note that this describes an ideal interaction between doctors and patients. The model obviously does not apply to chronic disease. Parsons' functionalist view (see Chapter 6) has also been criticized for its affirmation of the doctor's control function and for assuming lack of conflict between the roles of patients and doctors.

The patient's right to stay off work is an important constituent of the sick role. Obviously its performance varies with social and cultural context. On average, sick leave is shorter in Japan and America than in Europe; within countries, it is shorter in the private than in the public sector. Role performance depends also on economic factors. The rate of the workforce absence from work is higher during economic growth and lower in periods of recession and job insecurity.

Bureaucracy

Bureaucracy is a common phenomenon of large organizations, including health services. In Weber's view, bureaucratic organization is a consequence of increasing complexity in the division of labour (Weber 1958). Most people have come across the negative sides of bureaucracy. To understand how bureaucracy affects communication with patients you need to be aware of its main properties.

- *Hierarchy*. People engage in narrowly defined tasks and work under rules. Power is distributed according to defined areas of competence. Authority and responsibility are clearly defined for each member of staff. Doctors and nurses work in hierarchies with a number of different occupational roles oriented to different tasks.
- *Continuity*. The system is self-sustaining. Written records ensure machine-like accuracy, even if staff change. For example, shifts are not supposed to affect patient care.
- *Impersonality*. Work is done according to strict rules, without favouritism; officials are exchangeable. This gives officials the authority to act on behalf of the whole organization.
- *Expertise*. Officials are selected according to merit and are trained to have the necessary skills and knowledge to fulfil their function.

All this contributes to a rational organization of labour but it affects the interaction with patients negatively:

- the bureaucratic separation of tasks can result in fragmented care
- patients may receive contradictory signals from different encounters
- staff may develop stereotypical views of patients, judging their personality through the amount of work they cause.

Often you can observe an inverse relation between patient openness and position in the hierarchy: patients tend to talk more easily and more frankly to members of staff who occupy a lower position in the hierarchy, for example to cleaners, than to senior doctors and nurses.

The bureaucratic type of organization provides privileged social status and relative job security. It is often seen as the only means of providing services equally throughout a country.

Contemporary changes in the patient role

In many high income countries, the role of the patient is changing in several ways. These have been described by a British commentator, Angela Coulter (2002):

No longer is he or she simply a passive victim of illness. In the twenty-first century the patient is a decision-maker, care manager and co-producer of health, an evaluator, a potential change agent, a taxpayer and an active citizen whose voice must be heard by decision-makers. Acknowledging these roles and developing and extending active partnerships with patients has become essential for all health care providers, and in particular for those working on the front-line in primary care.

The key to restoring confidence lies as much in the hands of clinicians as it does in politicians. Clinicians could do a great deal to help inform and educate those who seek their help. If the public can be helped to understand the limits of medical care as well as its potential benefits, they are much more likely to use health services appropriately and responsibly. Recognition of the patient as an active, autonomous player in the health care system should have profound consequences for the way in which health care is delivered. Relationships between health professionals and the public they serve need to be transformed at all levels, organisational as well as individual ... Managers and clinicians will have to be prepared to cede some power and patients must be willing to take greater responsibility for their own health. These changes are necessary to ensure the sustainability of collective health care provision.

Summary

Good staff–patient communication is an important determinant of patient satisfaction and outcome of care. Various factors have been found to influence the style of interaction with patients. Research suggests that key aspects of a successful encounter include eliciting the full range of patients' concerns, showing empathy and delivering adequate information. Training of health professionals in interpersonal skills contributes to improvement of staff–patient interaction. The distribution of relative power in the staff–patient relationship is shaped by various factors, including cultural norms and the bureaucratic organization of health services.

References

Bernhart M, Wiadyana IGP, Wihardjo H, Pohan I (1999) Patient satisfaction in developing countries. *Social Science & Medicine* 48: 989–96.

Byrne PS, Long BEL (1976) *Doctors Talking to Patients: A Study of the Verbal Behaviour of GPs Consulting in Their Surgeries*. London: HMSO.

Chowdhury AM, Chowdhury S, Islam MN, Islam A and Vaughan LP (1997) Control of tuberculosis by community health workers in Bangladesh. *Lancet* 350: 169–72.

Clark JM (1981) Communication in nursing. *Nursing Times* January 1: 12–18.

Coulter A (2002) *The Autonomous Patient*. London: TSO.

Egbert L (1964) Reduction of post-operative pain by encouragement and instruction of patient. *New England Journal of Medicine* 270: 825–7.

Levinson W, Roter DL, Mullooly JP, Dull VT, Frankel RM (1997) Physician–patient communication: the relationship with malpractice claims among primary care physicians and surgeons. *Journal of the American Medical Association* 277: 553–9.

Nettleton S, Harding S (1994) Protesting patients: a study of complaints submitted to a Family Health Services Authority. *Sociology of Health & Illness* 16: 38–63.

Parsons T, Mayhew LH (eds) (1982) *On Institutions and Social Evolution. Selected Writings*. Chicago: University of Chicago Press.

Rusmiyati R (1997) Focus group discussions for developing a patient satisfaction questionnaire. Directorate of Health Center Development, Ministry of Health, Jakarta, Indonesia.

Sbaro JA, Sbaro JB (1994) Compliance and supervision of chemotherapy of tuberculosis. *Seminars in Respiratory Infections* 9: 120–7.

Silverman D (1984) Going private: ceremonial forms in a private oncology clinic. *Sociology* 18: 191–204.

Sinyor JK (1997) Pregnant women's satisfaction with antenatal care. Directorate of Health Center Development, Ministry of Health, Jakarta, Indonesia.

Strong PM (1979) *The Ceremonial Order of the Clinic*. London: Routledge & Kegan Paul.

U205 Course Team (1985). *Caring for Health. Dilemmas and Prospects*, Chapter 4. Milton Keynes: Open University Press.

Weber M (1958) Bureaucracy, in Gerth HH (ed. and trans.) *From Max Weber: Essays in Sociology*. Oxford: Oxford University Press.

Williams SJ, Calnan M (1991) Key determinants of consumer satisfaction with general practice. *Family Practice* 8: 237–42.

Public as consumers and policy makers

Overview

In the previous chapter you looked at the interpersonal relationship between staff and patients. This chapter examines the interaction of lay people, in their role as consumers and as members of communities, with health services. You will first explore the extent to which lay people can be thought of as consumers. You will then go on to consider the potential roles they might play in policy making, who should be consulted, and finally the different ways in which communities have been included.

Learning objectives

After working through this chapter, you will be better able to:

- outline the concept of consumerism in health services
- give examples of initiatives strengthening consumer power and community participation in health care
- discuss the ways in which the public can be involved in health care policy making.

Key terms

Community participation A process by which individuals or groups assume responsibility for health matters of their community.

Consumerism A social movement promoting and representing user interests in health services.

Consumerism

Consumerism is a movement that has appeared in many high and middle income countries since the 1960s, to protect consumer interests in private business relations. It extended later to public services, including health care. The underlying view is that providers tend to disregard consumer interests and therefore consumers' rights need to be protected. Provider power needs to be balanced by consumers who actively monitor and evaluate health services and who make informed choices.

In turn, giving people choice, for example between different providers, is thought to improve the quality of services and people's satisfaction. Consumer power is also seen to improve the responsiveness to complaints and strengthen people's rights. In this concept, health care is regarded as being just like any other service, a commodity that can be produced and consumed. But is that true?

Activity 11.1

To think about this question, compare consumer power in an interaction between a nurse and patient, and between a seller and buyer of a car. Jot down the similarities and differences, before comparing your thoughts with the feedback below.

Feedback

The power of a car buyer depends on information. The key mechanism of consumer power is choice. If provided with the necessary information on the car market, consumers can choose between several models and car dealers. But the buyer may not have information as complete as the seller may have, an advantage that might be exploited.

In health care, consumer sovereignty is reduced due to the uncertainty of type and amount of care needed. Health care workers act as *agents*, deciding on behalf of people the type and amount of care that is to be consumed. Health care is usually paid indirectly through insurance contributions or taxation. Unlike the car deal, it is not paid at the time of use, and those who pay may be different from those who actually consume.

Consumerism appears to be the vehicle for different political interests (Lupton 1997). The discourse on consumerism has been adopted both by community groups focusing on patient autonomy and policy makers favouring a free market model of health care. Therefore you need to be cautious as to the different motives of the actors advocating consumerism.

Choice and community empowerment

As you have seen, the analogy of health care and consumption of commercial goods is limited. However, increasingly there is choice in:

- logistical matters (e.g. choice of doctors and hospitals)
- clinical matters (e.g. deciding between treatment alternatives)
- political matters (e.g. local participation in decision making).

The extent of choice varies widely. In a number of countries health systems have responded to political demands and introduced various forms of public participation. Important, too, is defining and implementing people's rights. Political participation is part of a larger concept of community empowerment, a topic addressed further below (Saltman 1994).

First, though, it is important that you are aware of the different degrees of power available to patients. The following framework (based on Arnstein 1966) describes the spectrum of possibilities, ranging from the traditional position in which the patient displays little power and is largely 'manipulated' by the health care professional through to a situation in which the patient takes control:

manipulation – information – consultation – participation – partnership – control

Initiatives to strengthen consumer power

A number of initiatives have strengthened consumer powers in health services (Saltman and Figueras 1997). These involve:

- better information
- complaints-handling systems
- representation of consumers at various levels of health services
- mechanisms protecting patients' rights.

The protection of patients' rights has been approached in two main ways: charters setting out entitlements and expectations, and laws. The former is the approach adopted in the UK, where health care providers have developed explicit standards that patients can expect to receive. Here is an example of one from the main hospital in Cambridge:

- Care for every person with consideration and respect of their personal needs and wishes.
- Try to keep to appointment times and explain the reasons if we cannot.
- Explain any planned care and treatment (including any particular risks and their consequences) and obtain patients' permission before giving any treatment.
- Give straightforward and honest answers to any questions about their illness, treatment or care.
- Make sure that information about a patient is not passed on without their permission, except to other staff directly involved in their treatment and care.
- Explain to people that Cambridge is a teaching district for both medical students and nurses. Medical students may be attached to the team that is caring for a person. If the patient does not want this involvement, they have a right to say so and their wish will, of course, be respected.
- Deal promptly and sensitively with any complaints and apologize where appropriate.

In contrast to the charter approach, other countries have defined patient's rights by law. Finland introduced legislation in 1993 which gives the patients' ombudsman an important role in monitoring and implementing all matters concerning patient rights. The Netherlands have introduced legally defined patient rights and enhanced the provisions to enforce those rights through courts. There is also formalized participation of consumers in the decision making process of health care. In India, the government extended the Consumer Protection Act to private health services to ensure that patients receive appropriate quality of care. The objective was to provide a less costly remedy to consumer complaints than the more expensive civil litigation (Bhat 1996).

Has consumerism changed the heath care encounter?

There is no doubt that consumerism has been influential in challenging health care professions and increasing users' power. But have these political processes also changed the health care encounter? You would expect that the patient in the role of consumer would refuse paternalism and professional dominance and actively assess and, if necessary, counter, expert knowledge. Obviously the encounter is more complex. Deborah Lupton, an Australian researcher, has pointed out that seeing patients as consumers underestimates the cultural and emotional features that influence the staff-patient relationship. The feeling of dependency is central to the illness experience and may work against taking up a consumerist position. Illness, pain and disability tend to encourage a need for trust in experts and faith in health care. From her studies in Australia, there is evidence that the role patients take depends on their personal circumstances. In the health care encounter, patients may both pursue the ideal type 'active consumer' or 'passive patient' position, simultaneously or variously, depending on the context (Lupton 1997). As you saw in Chapter 10, the role of the patient is changing, at least in high income countries.

Public input into health care policy making

The following edited extract from an article by Jonathan Lomas, a Canadian health services researcher, focuses on the types of decision for which there is a potential role for public input into publicly funded health services.

 Activity 11.2

As you read it, make notes about the author's attitude to the following:

1   The reason why formal carers and policy makers are interested in lay involvement.
2   The reasons why policy makers need to be cautious in their expectations of lay involvement in the three key areas of decisions about funding, service provision and rationing.

 Reluctant rationers: public input to health care priorities

Collective health care decisions and public input

It is no coincidence that public interest in public involvement in health care decisions has occurred at the same time as concern about the ability of the state to continue to fund ever higher levels of service. Health care system providers and managers, as well as their public funders, are faced with increasingly tough and painful choices in the allocation of resources within and/or to the health care system. Not surprisingly, they are looking to share some of this pain with the public. The desire of governments, managers and providers for public input is, therefore, largely instrumental; they do not see public involvement as a goal in itself. These decision-makers wish to find ways to have the public take (or at least share) ownership of the tough choices they face in allocating increasingly scarce resources . . .

From this perspective there are certain expectations of public involvement: first, that representative individuals are willing and feel able to be involved – unwilling participants are unlikely to take or share ownership in the eventual decisions; second, that the public accepts the need to ration within a fixed public budget for health care – the alternative merely posits more resources as the solution; third, that mechanisms are available to ensure that public input generates representative views – this not being the case, a false 'public' imprimatur is placed on the lobbying positions of over-represented interests such as particular disease groups or health care employees; fourth, the public will not over-ride unambiguous information on the ineffectiveness of various service options – ignoring such data leads to less 'health' being produced for the same funds; and finally, that members of the public are willing and able to adopt a collective view rather than a self-interested view – allocation of public resources for health care is more about what communities need than about what individuals want . . .

Defining essential or core services, prioritisation, or rationing are three of the most common phrases used to describe the gradual transformation of implicit rules into explicit processes for resource allocation. Many countries have involved the public to some degree. The most publicised has been the Oregon process. Unfortunately, this exercise in democratic rationing provides few lessons about methodologies for collective decision-making (it was about the non-poor allocating health care resources for the poor), or those considering the breadth of possible public input to health care decisions (it addressed only public input to specific services that should be offered).

Table 11.1 outlines six questions under three types of collective decision-making for which there is a potential role for the public . . . The majority of reported exercises have tended to start out with a primary focus on question 4, motivated by the apparent need to limit

Table 11.1 Six collective health care decisions for which there is a potential role for public input

Type of decision	Specific question	Role
Service funding	1. Funding level What should be the level of public funding for the provision of health care services? 2. Funding arrangements Under what financing and organisational arrangements should services be offered?	Taxpayer
Services to offer	3. Broad service categories What broad categories of service should be offered as part of the publicly funded health care system? 4. Specific services What specific services should be offered within each broad category of publicly funded health care?	Collective decision-maker
Who should receive services?	5. Clinical circumstances What are the clinical circumstances of patients who should receive specific offered services? 6. Socio-demographic circumstances What are the socio-demographic circumstances of patients who should receive specific offered services?	Patient perspective

Source: Lomas (1997).

the service package available to the public within a jurisdiction. The complexity of the task has, however, driven most of these exercises back to question 3 . . .

The purpose of Table 11.1 is not, however, just to point out the limited nature of current exercises. Rather, it is to show that not only do individuals think as three persons within one – taxpayer with views about funding, collective decision-maker with opinions about services offered and patient with preferences about services received – but also that the system would *require* him or her to think in three different ways if he or she were to contribute comprehensively to health care decision-making.

Decisions on public funding

. . . As taxpayers, individuals appear to support increased funding for health care, at the expense of almost all other areas of public expenditure . . . From governments' current perspective of expenditure reductions, public input on the level of funding for health care may, therefore, be best left unsought.

. . . Our own research in Canada found that the average citizen was not interested in being involved in these funding decisions . . . These were decisions deemed appropriate for politicians and the experts. Furthermore, few individuals are interested in how the state chooses to pay its providers or organize the system; they are principally concerned about getting to see a provider when they want one.

Decisions on what services to offer under public funding

The second category of decision-making – what services to offer – is where public input to priority setting has focused most. The limits on public funding are, in this case, achieved by rationing services. Although many exercises have failed to make it explicit, the presumed role for individuals is as collective decision-makers, i.e. to decide not what services they personally wish to see offered but rather what services they believe would best serve the general community good. The overall level and arrangement of funding, whether decided via public input or not, is obviously the constraining influence.

If the task of priority setting is done at the level of broad service categories, such as 'nursing care', 'services for acute emergencies', 'preventive care' and so on, it appears that the public are at least able to provide reasonably consistent relative priorities. This approach was reflected in the 1994 World Bank Report with the recommendation that public funding should be reserved for essential services, defined with community input, and oriented in developing countries towards 'primary care'.

Average citizens are, however, largely reticent about their ability to perform this collective decision-maker role . . . in Canada two-thirds of individuals did not want to take responsibility for priority setting. Once the collective decision making turns to priorities amongst *specific* services such as types of surgery, treatment for addictions, specific diagnostic tests and so on, both the consistency of responses and the willingness of individuals to participate decline even further . . .

This is hardly surprising given the information needs. Focusing on a specific service invites consideration of its costs and benefits in precise terms; this is information that is often either not available or not readily understandable to the average citizen. The more specific the service over which citizens are being asked to pass a priority judgement, the more they are driven to want to know its costs and benefits for specific clinical and social circumstances. In the absence of such information, the public is being asked to do the logically absurd task of judging need (and, hence, priority) independently of patient circumstance . . .

Decisions on who should receive offered services

The third category of decisions is the specific circumstances of patients who should receive particular services, once it has been established that the services will be offered. In this case, restrictions on public funding relate to rationing among patients not services. Denying access to services offered under public funding, whether because of clinical or socio-demographic characteristics of a patient, has become a contentious element of many health care systems, potentially resulting in legal challenge. The contentious and sharply distributive nature of these questions takes us into the realm of moral philosophy.

. . . Using practice guidelines, some jurisdictions have put much (probably misplaced) faith in this approach to limiting the growth of medical services. Although in some cases these clinical considerations can be relatively straightforward, more often than not the task is technically challenging and demanding of expertise. It is not clear that there is any substantial role for public input to these expert decisions.

This is probably not true, however, for the socio-demographic characteristics of patients which might limit access to offered services. Factors such as age and lifestyle have either been used or come under consideration for use as ways of excluding some patients from receiving publicly funded services . . . Interestingly, in explicit exercises members of the public appear to be more willing than physicians and managers to ration services on the basis of such socio-demographic characteristics.

. . . [The] involvement of members of the public is politically advisable given the sensitive nature of decisions to deny patients access to services on the basis of their age, lifestyle or social circumstance. One would hope, however, that final decisions on such denials of access to services would not allow public views to over-ride existing protections for minorities, the disabled, or others, embodied within human rights legislation.

 Feedback

1 To share some of the pain of making hard choices with the public.

2 As regards public involvement in funding decisions, they generally want to increase spending on health care despite governments' desire to control spending; for decisions as to what services to provide, the public often feel ill equipped and reluctant to be involved; and the public find the task of rationing (at the level of individual patients) too technically challenging, though no such reluctance exists if the decisions are limited to sociodemographic factors such as age or sex.

An example of the latter comes from a survey carried out by Ann Bowling in the mid-1990s in which she sought the views of a large nationally representative sample of adults on priorities for health services (Bowling 1996). An interview survey based on a random sample of people aged 16 and over in Great Britain was undertaken. The response rate to the survey was 75%, and the total number of adults interviewed was 2005. Respondents were asked to prioritize 12 services. In addition, their attitudes to who should set priorities and allocate budgets were sought. The results showed that the highest priority was accorded to 'treatments for children with life threatening illness', and the next highest priority was accorded to 'special care and pain relief for people who are dying'. The lowest priorities were given to 'treatment for infertility' and 'treatment for people aged 75 and over with life threatening illness'. Most respondents thought that surveys like this one should be used in the planning of health services. Bowling concluded that the public prioritize treatments specifically for younger rather than older people and there is some public support for people with self-inflicted conditions (e.g. through smoking) receiving lower priority for care.

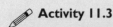 **Activity 11.3**

Despite Lomas's concerns about the role of the public in making policy about which services should be provided, numerous attempts have been made to involve them in this way. A review by Crawford *et al.* (2002) of the published accounts of such efforts in the UK, USA, Canada, Sweden and Australia found little evidence that involving the public (limited to patients in this case) had led to improvements in the quality of health care. As you read the following extract from their paper, note the three reasons the authors give to be cautious in interpreting these findings as discouraging.

📖 Systematic review of involving patients in the planning and development of health care

A review of more than 300 papers on involving patients in the planning and development of health care found that . . . involving patients has contributed to changes to services. The effects of involvement on accessibility and acceptability of services or impact on the satisfaction, health, or quality of life of patients has not been examined. . . . [A] potential problem in interpreting the results is that publication bias may favour the publication of reports from initiatives that were judged to be successful.

Several factors may account for our central finding, the limited amount of information about the effects of involving patients. The aims of involving patients have always been broader than just improving the quality of health care. Involving patients has been viewed by many as a democratic or ethical requirement: because patients pay for services they have a right to influence how they are managed. An alternative view is that involving patients is not intended to devolve power to patients but to legitimise the decisions of policy makers and administrators. It is argued that through consulting with users of health services, support for decisions that would otherwise be unpopular can be obtained. Such aims imply that establishing mechanisms for involving patients should be seen as an end in itself rather than as a means of improving the quality of services. However, initiatives that fall short of bringing about changes to services are not in keeping with the aims of current policy or patients.

The effects of involving patients are likely to be complex, affecting different aspects of services in different ways. The views of patients are among many factors that influence change in health services, and providers of health care remain the final arbiter of how much weight is attached to patients' views. Separating out change specifically attributable to the participation of patients is a difficult task. . . . Patients' involvement is not without its costs, and including outcome measures in future evaluations of involving patients could enable comparisons of different approaches and evaluation of the effects of suggestions made by patients.

. . . This absence of evidence should not be mistaken for an absence of effect. Health care providers may be increasingly required to demonstrate that they involve patients in the planning process, but they will also continue to be accountable for the decisions they make.

 Feedback

The three reasons suggested are as follows:

1 Improvement in health care is not the only objective of involving the public. Other worthy objectives are to be as democratic as possible and to gain public ownership of hard decisions. The achievement of these objectives should also be considered.

2 It is difficult to separate the effect of public involvement from other influences on decisions.

3 Absence of evidence is not the same as absence of effect.

The potential benefits of greater public involvement have been explained by two British commentators, Dominique Florin and Jennifer Dixon (2004).

 Public involvement in health care

Advocates of increased public involvement argue that public services are paid for by the people and therefore should be shaped more extensively by them, preferably by a fully representative sample. One assumption made is that greater public involvement will lead to more democratic decision making and, in turn, better accountability, but neither is necessarily the case. A second assumption is that more public involvement is an intrinsic good. This belief is based on values or ideology and thus cannot be tested, but it is often allied to beliefs that can be tested empirically. For example, one associated belief is that as many healthcare issues have important ethical as well as technical dimensions, involving the public may help ensure health policy decisions better reflect the values of the community. This belief could be tested by assessing how far the mechanisms for involving the public help to reach a generally accepted view on an ethical dilemma.

A second argument for increasing public involvement is that it will make services more responsive to the individuals and communities who use them and that more responsive services will lead to improved health. Underpinning these assumptions is the belief that professional definitions of benefit in health care can be at best only partial; only the users or local communities themselves know what they need, and it is ultimately their assessment of benefit that matters.

The second main issue raised by Lomas was which members of the public should be consulted. You have seen one approach (Bowling 1996) – surveys of large, randomly selected samples of the population. For many countries, the expense of such an approach has led to the exploration of other methods. One example was to see if the views of community leaders could substitute for more widespread consultation. Obinna Onwujekwe *et al.* (1999) compared the views of community leaders in three areas of Nigeria with the views of local people regarding the financing and distribution of drugs to treat onchocerciasis (river blindness). They found that while there was no significant difference in relation to the method of collecting payments, managing and making payments, who should set the level of payments and the drug distribution mechanisms, there were differences concerning how the scheme should be supervised.

Their conclusion was as follows.

Can community leaders' preferences be used to proxy those of the community as a whole?

It appears that one can never completely substitute preferences elicited from households with those of community leaders, as there are likely to be some points of disagreement between the two classes of people. However, bearing time and resource constraints in mind, one approach would be to collect information from community leaders during surveys and then discuss the results in general assemblies of communities, so that areas of conflict could be resolved before programme implementation.

The findings also show the importance of conducting a comparative analysis in different areas of the preferences of both community leaders and heads of households before mounting community-based health care interventions. Such an approach should help to discover whether, and if so where, there are disparities between the views of community leaders and heads of households and whether these vary between areas, in order to resolve any differences during the planning stage of any initiative. It is now well established from other research that people's own words and experiences bring into sharp focus the problems that influence their satisfaction with health care, and that addressing these problems by allowing community voices to be heard and affirming the importance of their experience for health care planning is essential in ensuring that widely available and efficacious primary health care interventions become effective in practice.

Summary

Various initiatives have been designed to transfer power to users of health services. They have involved better information, improvement of complaints handling, advocacy schemes, representation of consumers at various levels of health services and mechanisms protecting patients' rights. In this chapter you have examined the relevance of consumerism to health care and the ways in which the public might be more involved in policy making.

References

Arnstein SR (1966) A ladder of citizen participation. *American Institute of Planners Journal* 35: 216–24.

Bhat R (1996) Regulating the private health care sector: the case of the Indian consumer protection act. *Health Policy and Planning* 11: 265–79.

Bowling A (1996) Health care rationing: the public's debate. *British Medical Journal* 312: 670–4.

Crawford MJ, Rutter D, Manley C, Waver T, Bhui K, Fulop N, Tyrer P (2002) Systematic review of involving patients in the planning and development of health care. *British Medical Journal* 325: 1263–8.

Florin D, Dixon J (2004) Public involvement in health care. *British Medical Journal* 328: 159–61.

Lomas J (1997) Reluctant rationers: public input to health care priorities. *Journal of Health Services Research & Policy* 2: 103–11.

Lupton D (1997) Consumerism, reflexivity and the medical encounter. *Social Science & Medicine* 45: 373–81.

Onwujekwe O, Shu E, Okonkwo P (1999) Can community leaders' preferences be used to proxy those of the community as a whole? *Journal of Health Services Research & Policy* 4: 133–8.

Saltman RB (1994) Patient choice and patient empowerment in northern European health systems: a conceptual framework. *International Journal of Health Services* 24: 210–29.

Saltman RB, Figueras J (eds) (1997) *European Health Care Reform: Analysis of Current Strategies.* Copenhagen: World Health Organization Regional Office for Europe.

World Bank (1994) *Investing in Health.* Washington, DC: World Bank.

SECTION 4

Outcome of health care

12 | Outcomes

Overview

Now that you have examined inputs and processes you will move on to look at the results of health care. The outcome of health care is the change (hopefully, improvement) in the health status of patients. In this chapter you will learn what aspects of a patient's health status should be measured, how health status can be measured, and the characteristics of a good measure.

Learning objectives

After working through this chapter you will be better able to:

- **define and describe health status measures (impairment, disability and quality of life)**
- **conceptualize the relationships between different dimensions of outcomes**
- **understand the difference between objective and subjective measures.**

Key terms

Disability (functional status) The impact on the patient's ability to function.

Disease-specific measures Instruments that focus on the particular aspects of the disease being studied.

Generic measures Instruments that measure general aspects of a person's health, such as mobility, sleeping and appetite.

Impairment The physical signs of the condition (pathology), usually measured by clinicians.

Quality of life (handicap or well-being) The impact of the condition on the social functioning of a person, partly determined by the person's environment.

Reliability The extent to which an instrument produces consistent results.

Responsiveness The extent to which an instrument detects real changes in the state of health of a person.

Validity The extent to which an instrument measures what it intends to measure.

What is outcome?

Outcome is a patient's health status after receiving a health care intervention (treatment). The effectiveness of health care is assessed by the impact it has on a patient's health. To do this, you need to compare their health status before with that after the intervention. This raises three questions:

- What aspect of a patient's health status should be measured?
- How can health status be measured?
- What is a good measure?

What aspect of a patient's health status should be measured?

This depends on what impact you expect the intervention to have. For example, if you expect the death rate from the condition to be reduced, it would be reasonable to consider mortality as an outcome. But mortality would be inappropriate if the intervention is expected to relieve pain only.

There are five aspects of health status to choose from when selecting appropriate outcomes to measure:

- death/survival
- impairment – the physical signs of the condition (pathology) usually measured by clinicians
- disability (also referred to as functional status) – the impact on the patient's ability to function
- quality of life (also referred to as handicap or well-being) – the impact of the condition on the social functioning of a person, partly determined by a person's environment
- satisfaction with outcome – as distinct from satisfaction with the humanity of the care received.

Impairment, disability and quality of life are related to one another. This can be seen best if you consider an example. A common problem among elderly men is that their prostate enlarges, causing several urinary symptoms such as having to urinate more frequently, including during the night when it disturbs their sleep. Figure 12.1 illustrates the relationship between the three aspects of health status.

Impairment refers to the effect the condition has on their physiology. In this case, because there is partial obstruction at the neck of the bladder, the rate at which a man can urinate is reduced (referred to as the urine flow rate). This can be detected by a clinician but it is not the reason that men present to their doctor. What they actually complain about is the effect the condition is having (the symptoms), such as having to go to the toilet frequently. Symptoms are the ways in which a condition disables or reduces a person's functional status. This needs to be distinguished from the third aspect, the impact that the condition has on a person's social functioning. How bothersome the symptoms are will vary between patients and depend to a considerable extent on the physical, social and psychological environment. If a man is a train driver and cannot easily leave the train cab to go to the toilet frequently, the condition will have a major impact as he may be unable to continue in

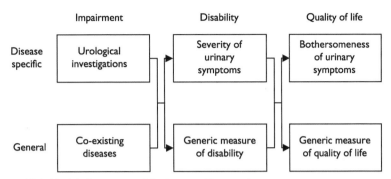

Figure 12.1 Model of measures of the impact of lower urinary tract symptoms

(Source: London School of Hygiene & Tropical Medicine staff)

his job. In contrast, going to the toilet frequently may be nothing more than a nuisance for an office worker.

Activity 12.1

How could the health status of someone with arthritis of the hip be assessed? You need to consider their impairment, disability and quality of life.

Feedback

You should have identified the following:

- Impairment could be assessed by a clinician examining the person in terms of the extent to which they can move their leg.
- Disability could be assessed in terms of how far they can walk without pain.
- Quality of life could be assessed in terms of the impact their disability is having on the activities they like to do, such as gardening, playing sports or shopping.

While these three aspects are related to one another, it isn't a straightforward relationship. The extent to which someone is disabled can be explained to some extent by their level of impairment. But research shows that only about 25% of a person's disability is 'explained' by their impairment. This is because people have considerable capacity to compensate and learn to accommodate their impairment. People learn ways of coping with impairment – the Paralympics are a shining example of how far some people can go to overcome impairment.

Similarly, disability does not automatically affect a person's quality of life. Only about 25% of a person's quality of life is explained by their level of disability. So, the man who has to visit the toilet every hour but loves going to the cinema will ensure he sits at the end of a row so he doesn't disturb others. Quality of life is affected by many things (such as housing, employment, relationships), not just health status. So it is not surprising that health status has only a partial influence on quality of life.

How can health status be measured?

The measurement of mortality is obvious and straightforward, though in high income countries in recent years there have been debates about how death is defined – the moment at which the heart and lungs stop functioning or when the brain stops functioning? The development of life-support technology that can maintain a person's breathing has raised medical and ethical questions about the distinction between dead and alive.

Measurement of the four other aspects of health status requires a mixture of clinician and patient involvement. *Impairment* is generally assessed by a clinician and involves the objective measurement of a person's body. It may focus on such things as the person's physiology, biochemistry or immune status. It usually involves the use of a measuring device. This may be quite simple – for example, weighing scales and a tape measure to determine how well a child is growing. Increasingly, particularly in high income countries, it involves expensive high technology equipment such as MRI scanners.

In contrast, *disability* may be assessed by clinicians or patients. Clearly some symptoms, such as pain, can only be detected and 'measured' by patients. But others, such as the distance a patient can walk or the weight a person can lift, can be either assessed by a patient or observed by a clinician.

Quality of life is, by definition, a subjective assessment of how a person's state of health is affecting them socially and psychologically. The only person who can assess this is the person themselves. You may have a view of the quality of someone else's life, but it may differ markedly from that person's self-assessment. A common example is that of someone confined to a wheelchair. Able-bodied observers may feel that the person's quality of life is poor, but that is a view almost certainly not supported by the affected person.

Satisfaction with the outcome is, like quality of life, inherently a personal view. Some people may be satisfied with a modest improvement in their symptoms, whereas someone else may be disappointed and only be satisfied if the symptoms have gone completely.

A key distinction, which you may have identified, is whether the aspect of health being assessed involves subjective or objective measures. These are often confused with whether or not the measurement can be 'trusted'. People often assume that objective measures are 'better' than subjective. This is incorrect. Whichever type of measure you use, you need to know how accurate it is.

What is a good measure?

A good measurement instrument must be valid and reliable. It is *valid* if it measures what it intends to measure. It is *reliable* if it produces consistent results.

There are two ways in which reliability can be tested. If two or more people use the measure, do they get the same answer? This is as important a consideration for doctors interpreting an X-ray (do they all see the same things?) as it is for two people interviewing a patient about their quality of life. This is known as inter-observer (or inter-rater) reliability. You also want to know that if a measuring instrument is used again on the same patent you will get the same answer (assuming the patient's health hasn't altered between the two assessments). This known as intra-observer reliability.

There is a third aspect you need to consider when assessing the impact of health care – the *responsiveness* of the instrument to change: can the instrument detect meaningful changes?

Finally, you need to consider when to assess the impact of a health care intervention. Too short an observation period may render false results.

 Activity 12.2

When do you think it would be appropriate to assess the outcome of the following interventions?

1 Measles immunization
2 Hip surgery
3 Treatment of cerebral malaria
4 Anti-smoking posters.

 Feedback

You should have suggested the following times, approximately:

1 Several years, as the aim of immunization is to prevent measles throughout childhood.

2 About 6 months to see any improvement in mobility. Any earlier, the patient may not yet have recovered fully from their operation or completed their rehabilitation so you might underestimate the benefit of the operation. You might also have suggested about 10 years if you are interested in the commonest long term problem, that of loosening of the hip prosthesis.

3 Several days, since if the treatment is going to be successful it will take effect fairly quickly.

4 Several weeks, because if the posters are going to have any impact it will be soon after they are put up. If you leave the assessment any longer, any short term benefit might have disappeared as people take-up smoking again.

 Activity 12.3

The distinction between subjective and objective measures is often confused with the issue of the validity and reliability of a measure. This is addressed in the following edited essay by Paul Cleary (1997), an expert in health status measurement.

As you read it, make notes on why subjective measures should be included when assessing people's health state.

Subjective and objective measures of health: which is better when?

Clinicians and biomedical researchers frequently question the value of subjective measures of health. Whether a measure is subjective (based on individual awareness or experience) or objective (existing and measurable, independent of individual experiences) certainly is an important characteristic of variables related to health states. However, it is my experience that participants in such debates often confuse the distinction between variable type and measurement strategy. For example, some researchers are uncomfortable with the results of surveys about health-related quality of life and would prefer to use only data derived from medical record reviews for their analyses. It is important to understand both the inherent characteristics of the variables we are interested in and the strengths and weaknesses of different measurement strategies if we are to obtain the best possible data for health and health services studies . . .

Which aspects of health should be measured depends on the hypotheses being tested. For example, if the hypothesis is that a particular dietary supplement will increase the number of red cells in the blood, then measures of symptoms, difficulty performing basic activities of daily living, or general health perceptions are probably not needed . . . If, however, one wants to assess the impact of improving the red cell concentration on patients' lives, it would be important to measure aspects of health-related quality of life, such as fatigue and functional status . . .

Subjective measures can sometimes also provide accurate and efficient assessments of objective states. Physical functioning is such a variable. Patients can be asked whether they have difficulty going up and down stairs, or an observer can visit their homes to observe whether they can or cannot climb stairs. This is a situation in which objective measures are available and can be more reliable and valid, if properly administered, than patient self-reports, but such methods are often prohibitively expensive. Extensive research in this area has led to the development of short, functional status measures that can be administered directly to patients very efficiently and which have excellent reliability and validity. Thus, the use of such subjective measures is now widely accepted.

Probably the most subjective concept in health status assessment is perceived health. A typical question used to assess this variable is: 'Overall, how would you rate your health?' Respondents usually are then provided with a five-point Likert scale (poor, good, very good, excellent) or a 0–10 rating scale on which they can rate their health. To those trained in physical or biological sciences, this type of measure may seem problematic. What exactly does this variable measure? How can one possibly interpret such a subjective impression?

This measure is known to mean different things to different people and, in some ways, that is its strength. We view general health perception as an individual's synthesis of various objective and subjective information about health that integrates this information using individual weights and preferences. Whether this is a good thing to measure is partly a matter of opinion, but it is also an empirical issue . . . The empirical question is whether such a measure provides information that other variables do not, and/or whether it reliably predicts phenomena of interest.

One of the most compelling reasons for assessing general perceived health is that it predicts subsequent morbidity and mortality, even after controlling for other biological and health status variables. For example, self-evaluations of health predict mortality, even after statistically controlling for the presence of health problems, disability, and/or other risk factors. It has been found that elderly people with perceived poor health were six times as likely to die in a 4-year period than those who reported that their health was excellent – a relative risk greater than that for smoking (Idler and Kasl 1991).

We do not fully understand why perceived health is such a good predictor of mortality. There may be other unmeasured objective measures of health that could reduce the residual explanatory predictive power of perceived health. However, considering the sophistication of available studies, the power of this variable is striking. Several reasons why this variable predicts mortality have been posited. It may reflect a self-fulfilling prophecy. That is, people who think they are in poor health may not protect and promote their health as much as other people. Another explanation is that such ratings may capture more information than is available in other types of assessments. When individuals rate their health, they may consider family, genetic and health history information, information about their physical and social environment, and their own attitudes and expectations about health, in addition to numerous signs and symptoms related to their health. People may use their knowledge and experience to provide a more integrated and informative rating than is possible with other variables typically available to researchers. Irrespective of which explanation is correct, data on the relationships between mortality rates and subjective states such as chest pain or general health perception should put to rest any qualms about the value of subjective measures of health.

Some researchers are uncomfortable with subjective variables because they are perceived as unreliable. Such people often think of data from medical records as 'hard' data, whereas they think of survey responses as 'soft' data. Thus, rather than judging the relative theoretical value of objective and subjective measures, some researchers' selection of variables is unduly influenced by their negative opinions about the value of survey data relative to other types of information . . .

Even though symptoms are inherently subjective, some researchers seem to feel more comfortable using medical record notations, rather than information from patient surveys, as symptom measures. However, a measure of chest pain collected using a standardized instrument, such as the Rose questionnaire, using rigorous sampling and survey administration techniques, will yield a measure that is more reliable and valid than indications in medical records that were collected using different techniques by many clinicians who had their own subjective impressions of how 'sick' an individual patient was.

Many 'objective' or partly objective variables, such as functional status, probably are best measured using objective methods. However, it is important to recognize that abstracting such information from medical records does not mean that it is 'objective'. Medical records frequently contain functional assessments that were obtained by health care professionals with no training in standardized measurement and that are largely subjective measures. Such variables may be measured more efficiently, reliably and validly with standardized subjective measures.

Many clinical, health services and health policy studies test hypotheses based on subjective variables. We need to learn a great deal more about individual variations in how people perceive, interpret and report subjective states such as symptoms and general health perception. Nevertheless, concern about reliability and validity, although always an overriding research consideration, should not preclude considerations of subjective variables since extensive methodological research on the measurement of such variables has led to techniques that allow researchers to measure them with a level of reliability and validity that frequently exceeds the assessment of objective states. The types of variables to be assessed in any given study should be determined on the basis of the hypotheses being tested, not on poorly founded opinions about the value of different data collection strategies.

 Feedback

Subjective measures may:

1 be the appropriate aspect to be assessed, for example if the treatment is intended to improve a patient's quality of life.

2 provide a more efficient means of assessing an objective state, for example a mailed self-completed questionnaire is a cheaper way of ascertaining how far someone can walk than sending an observer to visit them.

3 provide more valid assessment of a person's health state and prognosis.

4 provide more reliable assessment as new data using standard definitions may be used whereas 'objective' data in medical records are dependent on the definitions used by each and every clinician recording the information.

Which measure to use?

Apart from selecting a measure that is valid, reliable and responsive, what other issues should you consider in choosing a measure? One consideration is between *generic* and *disease-specific measures.*

Generic measures, as the term implies, measure general aspects of health rather than those aspects that are particularly affected by the disease being studied. The most widely used generic measure is the Short Form 36 (SF36), so-called because it contains 36 questions (or items). It covers both disability and quality of life. The 36 items cover eight dimensions: physical functioning; role limitations due to physical problems; bodily pain; general health perception; energy/vitality; social functioning; role limitations due to emotional problems; and mental health.

The advantage of using a generic, rather than disease-specific, measure is that you can then compare the benefit that patients with disease X gain from treatment with the benefit gained by patients with disease Y. The disadvantage is that because it is generic, several dimensions being measured may not be affected by the disease or treatment so they are not 'responsive'. As a result, generic measures may not be sensitive enough to detect and quantify the effect of an intervention.

In contrast, disease-specific measures are designed to be appropriate for a particular disease. For example, a measure for assessing hip replacement surgery would focus on the amount of hip pain and mobility – the two principal areas in which you should see an improvement. The advantage is that disease-specific measures are highly responsive. The disadvantage is that you cannot compare the benefits of hip surgery with that of, say, malaria treatment.

Many generic and disease-specific measures have been developed. Lists of those available can be found in books and on the Internet. When choosing which to use you should ensure that its validity and reliability have been rigorously tested and shown to be good.

The other consideration is whether you measure the *final outcome* or an *intermediate outcome*. The final outcome is what you are trying to achieve by intervening. For example, a measles immunization programme aims to reduce child deaths from measles. Therefore, to assess using the final outcome, you would need to wait perhaps 10 years and measure the mortality from measles in a cohort of children who were the target of the immunization programme. However, governments, health services and the public might want to know what effect the programme is having sooner than that. What you could do is use an intermediate outcome, such as the level of uptake of immunization, which would be known within a year or so. Strictly speaking, an immunization rate is a measure of process (or activity) and not outcome. Its use as an indication of outcome is only justifiable because it is well established that immunizing a child will reduce or eliminate its risk if contracting measles. It can therefore be assumed that a high immunization rate will result in fewer deaths.

Summary

People's state of health can be assessed in terms of impairment, disability and quality of life. In addition, you can measure their level of satisfaction with their outcome. Any measure, whether subjective or objective, must be valid, reliable and responsive. You should also consider whether or not to use generic or disease-specific measures, or both. Many such measures have been developed and ones that have been properly tested and evaluated should be selected. Devising a new measure is a complex, time-consuming process and should only be considered if no suitable measure exists.

References

Cleary PD (1997) Subjective and objective measures of health: which is better when? *Journal of Health Services Research & Policy* 2: 3–4.

Idler EL, Kasl S (1991) Health perceptions and survival: do global evaluations of health status really predict mortality? *Journal of Gerontology* 46: S55–65.

SECTION 5

Organization of services

13 | Analysing health systems

Overview

In previous sections you were introduced to health services and focused on inputs, processes and outcomes. This section will give you an opportunity to explore the different methods used for international comparison of health systems. Chapter 14 provides an overview of the theory of state intervention in health care and describes some of the universal factors shaping the organization of health systems.

But first you will consider the value of studying health systems and the inherent dangers that await the unwary. You will then examine the strengths and weaknesses of the different methods of comparing health systems. Finally, you will consider an alternative approach to defining health care systems.

Learning objectives

After working through this chapter, you will be better able to:

- **suggest reasons why it is difficult to compare health services between countries**
- **outline the different approaches to health systems analysis**
- **give examples of root definitions based on the customers, actors, transformation, *Weltanschauung*, ownership and environment (CATWOE) elements.**

Key terms

CATWOE A mnemonic for customers, actors, transformation, *Weltanschauung*, ownership and environment – criteria for assessing a health care system.

Horizontal equity The equal treatment of individuals or groups in the same circumstances.

Macroeconomic efficiency The total costs of the health system in relation to overall health status; countries differ in how efficiently their health systems convert resources used into health gains.

Microeconomic efficiency The scope for achieving greater efficiency from existing resources; it is of two types – allocative and technical efficiency.

Multidimensional model An analytical approach integrating selected socioeconomic, cultural and organizational factors.

Root definition A description of a system based on each of the CATWOE (see above) elements.

Vertical equity The principle that individuals who are unequal should be treated differently according to their level of need.

Why study health systems?

Why should you study different health systems? What can you learn from international comparison?

 Activity 13.1

Thinking of your own country, how has health care been influenced by other countries' experience?

 Feedback

Medicine, nursing and health sciences are international. There is an active international dissemination of knowledge and technology. You may also have thought of international drug and supplies companies, textbooks and meetings. Educational and professional career structures may be similar between countries.

But what about health services organization and management? There are several reasons to learn lessons from other countries' health systems:

- It can provide *new perspectives* from which to view your own system.
- You may use international experience to *predict change* in your own country.
- You may use this information to establish *a general theory* of health services to help you better understand some of the universal problems of health care and help develop possible solutions.

You need to be aware, however, that there are a number of dangers in international comparison.

1 *Complexity* – health systems are extremely complex. Though they have common features, they are strikingly different. You need only imagine the potentially infinite number of interrelationships between inputs, processes and outcomes.

2 *Pluralism* – there is a plurality of systems in most countries. It is not unusual for a country to have a private, a tax-funded and a social insurance-based subsystem within the health sector.

3 *Definitions* – international variations in inputs can be explained by varying definitions of, for example, nurses or hospitals.

4 *Environment* – each system is influenced by its political, economic and cultural environment.

5 *Information* – there are large gaps in available information.

Approaches to comparing health systems

Systematic country comparisons have been performed since the 1960s. Note that the conceptual framework of analysis has changed over time from simple classifications to more sophisticated approaches. You should be aware of three methods, which reflect increasing levels of complexity.

- *Ideal types* (see Chapter 6) – these are hypothetical models highlighting certain features that may have explanatory power. For example, you may compare the ideal type description of a social insurance scheme to the actual implementation in countries.
- *Multidimensional models* – this approach integrates selected aspects of health systems, such as social, economic or political factors. For example, you may investigate how universal factors such as urbanization, industrialization or technology affect the organization of health systems.
- *Systems analysis* – this approach provides an entire picture of a health system, which takes account of the different levels of complexity and the hierarchy of subsystems and wider systems.

 Activity 13.2

In the following article by two health economists, Anne Mills and Kent Ransom (2001) explore the strengths and weaknesses of the different ways of thinking about health systems. They also provide facts about different health systems and the ways in which some of them have changed. While reading, focus on the different ways of dealing with complexity and the advantages of a systems (or 'modular') approach. Consider the following questions:

1 What evidence is there that the health of a nation does not depend entirely on its economic performance?
2 How can health systems be described in order to throw light on their efficiency and equity?
3 How could you judge whether a system is equitable horizontally and vertically?

 The design of health systems

Health systems are the means whereby . . . programs and interventions . . . are planned and delivered. They are a crucial influence on the extent to which countries are able to address their disease burden and improve overall levels of health and the health of particular groups in the population.

A health system has been defined as 'the combination of resources, organisation, financing and management that culminate in the delivery of health services to the population' (Roemer 1991). Health systems vary greatly from country to country. Unlike the study of disease, there is little standardized terminology or methodology for studying and understanding health systems. Each country's health system is the product of a complex range of factors, not least historical patterns of development and the power of different interest groups. Nonetheless, it is possible to identify common features, and knowledge is increasing on what design features are associated with what outcomes, thus facilitating cross-country learning.

It is extremely important to study and understand how health systems function and how they can be changed. Total expenditure on health care was around 5.4% of world gross domestic product (GDP) in 1994, or 4.5% of the GDP of the low and middle income countries, which contain 84% of the world's population. Health services are thus one of the largest sectors in the world economy. However, countries at similar income levels differ greatly in how effectively they look after the health of their populations. The health-related differences between countries of similar income can be enormous, as shown in Figure 13.1. While a variety of factors affect health, it is clear that the health system is an important determinant.

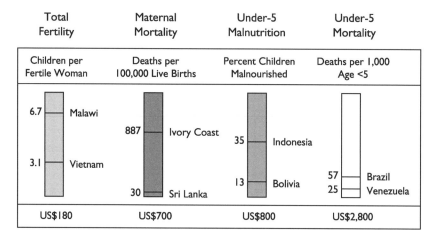

Approximate Income Levels (US$ per capita per year)

Figure 13.1 Outcomes at similar income levels (Mills and Ransom 2001)

Gro Harlem Brundtland, the director general of the WHO appointed in 1998, emphasized that 'in many parts of the world, health systems are ill equipped to cope with present demands, let alone those they will face in the future' and that 'there is a need to develop more effective health systems' (WHO 1999). Understanding health systems and how they can be changed is an endeavor that can benefit from the insights of a number of disciplines, most notably economics, sociology, anthropology, political science, and management science. In recent years, not least because concerns of resource scarcity, cost inflation, and efficiency have been uppermost in policy makers' minds, the discipline of economics has had a dominant influence on the study of health systems. We therefore draw primarily on economics to review key features of the design of health systems . . .

Since the seminal study of Kohn and White in 1976, an expanding body of literature has been attempting both to systematize the discussion of the various elements of health systems and to categorize health systems into a limited number of different types (Kohn and White 1976; Roemer 1991). These two issues are taken in turn.

Elements of health systems

Roemer (1991) identifies five major categories that enable a comprehensive description of a country's health system to be made (Figure 13.2):

• production of resources (trained staff, commodities such as drugs, facilities, knowledge)

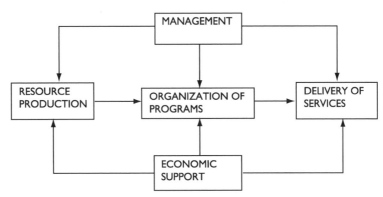

Figure 13.2 The elements of health systems (Mills and Ransom 2001)

- organization of programs (by government ministries, private providers, voluntary agencies)
- economic support mechanisms (sources of funds, such as tax, insurance, user fees)
- management methods (planning, administration, regulation, legislation)
- delivery of services (preventive and curative personal health services; primary, second-ary, and tertiary services; public health services; services for specific population groups, such as children, or for specific conditions, such as mental illness).

This categorization is helpful for describing health systems; indeed, Roemer applies it in his book to a very large number of countries. However, it is not helpful for understanding how health systems behave in terms of efficiency and equity. This would require much more detailed subcategories and greater elaboration of the relationships, not just within each category but particularly between categories (for example, between economic support mechanisms and organization of programs).

The Organization for Economic Cooperation and Developmcnt (OECD) has developed a categorization that is helpful for understanding not only the economic dimensions of health systems in OECD countries, but also the directions that reforms are taking them in (OECD 1992). The key categories are:

- whether the prime funding source consists of payments that are made voluntarily (as in private insurance or payment of user fees) or are compulsory (as in taxation or social insurance)
- whether services are provided by direct ownership (termed the integrated pattern, where a Ministry of Health or social insurance agency provides services itself), by contractual arrangements (where a Ministry of Health or social insurance agency con-tracts with providers to deliver services), or simply by private providers (paid by direct out-of-pocket payments)
- how services are paid for (prospectively, where financial risk is transferred to providers; or retrospectively, where the cost of care is reimbursed).

These various arrangements are explained further below in the relevant sections.

Typologies of health systems

In order to make comparisons of how different types of health system perform, it is necessary to group countries into a manageable number of types. There have been various attempts to do this. Countries can be classified according to:

- the dominant method of financing (for example, tax, social insurance, private insurance, out-of-pocket payments)
- the underlying political philosophy (for example, capitalist, socialist)
- the nature of state intervention (for example, to cover the whole population or only the poor)
- the level of gross national product (for example, low, middle, high)
- historical or cultural attributes (for example, industrialized, non-industrialized, transitional).

A key difficulty, however, is that countries do not fit neatly into these categories. Roemer, for example, uses two dimensions:

- economic level (with four categories: affluent and industrialized, developing and transitional, very poor, resource-rich)
- health system policies (again with four categories: entrepreneurial and permissive, welfare orientated, universal and comprehensive, socialist and centrally planned).

While some of these categories are less relevant than they were at the time (for example, centrally planned), it is also the case that the second dimension does not classify well the health systems of low- and middle-income countries, which tend to be fragmented, with different arrangements for different population groups. For example, Roemer classifies Thailand as 'entrepreneurial and permissive,' and Mexico and India as 'welfare orientated.' Yet, as shown in Table 13.1, which summarizes the structure of the health systems in these three countries plus Zambia, these four countries cannot be clearly categorized into such neat categories.

Since a typology suitable for low- and middle-income countries has yet to be worked out, we propose a simple framework (shown in Figure 13.3) that identifies four key actors:

1 the government or professional body that structures and regulates the system;
2 the population, including patients, who as individuals and households ultimately pay for the health system and receive services;
3 financing agents, who collect funds and allocate them to providers or purchase services at national or lower levels;

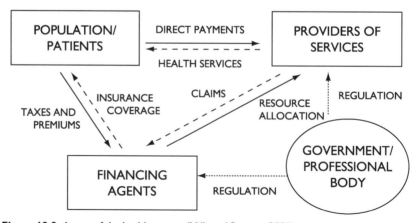

Figure 13.3 A map of the health system (Mills and Ransom 2001)

Table 13.1 Illustrations of the structure of health systems

Zambia (per capita GNP $380)

The health system is made up of a large public sector, covering all levels from primary to tertiary, which until recently has been very centralized. There is an extensive network of industrial (concentrated in urban areas) and mission (church) services (generally rural), subsidized by the state. Private doctors practice in the main cities, and there is a large informal sector of traditional practitioners and drug sellers. There are only a handful of private hospitals (0.2% of beds are in the private-for-profit sector and 25% in the mission sector). An executive agency has been created to take over management responsibility from the Ministry of Heath at national level, and the role of health districts has been strengthened.

India (per capita GNP $390)

The public sector is large in absolute terms, providing all levels of care. Health care is in general a state function, with central government involved mainly in overall policy and specific disease control programs. There is a large formal private sector, providing both ambulatory and inpatient care, and an even larger informal sector consisting of unlicensed and unqualified practitioners and drug sellers. There is limited formal interaction between public and private sectors. A compulsory state insurance system covers lower paid, formal-sector workers, and there is another scheme for government workers. There are numerous community-based health schemes, some with an insurance component.

Mexico (per capita GNP $3680)

Public and private sectors play an important role in financing and provision. The health sector is highly segmented. Formal sector employees (roughly 60% of the population) are covered by various social insurance institutions. The poor receive care through government facilities or private providers (allopathic and traditional). There is little interaction between public and private sectors, either in the form of regulation or contracting for service delivery. There is much duplication and waste of resources between the three 'sub-systems' – social security, other government, and private. Mexico's health sector reform plan is based on decentralization and managed-market ideas.

Thailand (per capita GNP $2800)

Both public and private sectors are large, providing all levels of care. There is widespread use of the private sector, especially for outpatient care. Different population groups have different rights to care, and there are an increasing number of public and private arrangements. Compulsory social insurance covers those in formal employment and finances care provided by public and private hospitals (chosen by the insured). Civil servants have their own medical benefit scheme that pays for care at public and private hospitals. A prepayment scheme (voluntary health care) is available in rural areas. The poor can obtain a low-income card, which exempts them from fees charged in public facilities.

Note: GNP is in 1997 prices

Source: Mills and Ransom (2001).

4   the providers of services, who themselves can be categorized in various ways, such as by level (primary, secondary, tertiary), function (curative, preventive), ownership (public; private, for-profit; private, not-for-profit), degree of organization (formal, informal), or medical system (allopathic, Ayurvedic).

and four key functions required in any health system:

*   regulation
*   financing (through taxes, premiums, and direct payments)
*   resource allocation
*   providing services.

Evaluation of health systems

The criteria frequently used to judge health systems are efficiency and equity. Efficiency has a number of different dimensions:

- Macroeconomic efficiency refers to the total costs of the health system in relation to overall health status; countries differ in how efficiently their health systems convert resources used into health gains.
- Microeconomic efficiency refers to the scope for achieving greater efficiency from existing resources. It is of two types:

  — allocative efficiency: devoting resources to that mix of activities that will have greatest impact on health (that is, is most cost-effective)
  — technical efficiency: using only the minimum necessary resources to finance, purchase, and deliver a particular activity or set of activities (that is, avoiding waste).

Equity refers to the distribution of the costs of health services and the benefits obtained from their use between different groups in the population. It is inherently a question of values; however, indicators of who pays for health services and who receives benefits provide evidence on the degree of equity achieved by particular health systems. Equity can be expressed in two different ways (Donaldson and Gerard 1993):

1 Horizontal equity refers to the equal treatment of equals. With respect to financing and resource allocation, this implies that the charge levied by all agents or providers for a particular good or service should be the same for households with equal ability to pay (regardless of gender, marital status, and so on). Horizontal equity is therefore assessed by the extent to which there is variation in contribution levels among those with similar ability to pay. With respect to provision, horizontal equity means that individuals with the same health condition should have equal access to health services.
2 Vertical equity is based on the principle that individuals who are unequal in society should be treated differently. Vertical equity in the financing and purchasing or health services means that consumers should be charged for the same good or service according to their ability to pay.

Table 13.2 demonstrates how equity and efficiency criteria can be used to set goals for the financing, allocation of resources, and provision of health services, and for evaluating their performance.

 Feedback

1 As is apparent from Figure 13.1, countries with similar wealth (measured by average income levels) differ in population health measures; for example, maternal mortality in Ivory Coast is almost 30 times as high as in Sri Lanka.

2 The OECD suggests that three factors need to be considered: the source(s) of funding for health care (see Chapter 7); the relationship between purchasers and providers; and how services are paid for.

3 Horizontal equity would be assessed by considering the extent to which people with similar needs are treated the same (equal treatment for equal need). Vertical equity is based on the principle that individuals who are unequal in society should be treated differently (unequal treatment for unequal needs).

Table 13.2 Equity and efficiency goals for the financing, purchasing and provision of health care

	Efficiency		Equity	
Functions	Allocative	Technical	Horizontal	Vertical
Financing	–	Maximize the proportion of resources raised that are actually available for purchasing health care (for example, reduce the overhead costs of collecting taxes)	Equal payment by those with equal ability to pay (for example, same insurance premium for same income group)	Payment in relation to ability to pay (for example, progressive income tax rates)
Allocating resources	Purchase that mix of interventions that provides the greatest health gains	Maximize the proportion spent by agents that are actually available for providing health care	Services purchased for similar groups (for example, the elderly) should be the same in different geographical areas	Services purchased should reflect the different needs of different groups (for example, the elderly versus children)
Providing services	Provide those interventions that return the greatest value for money (for example, in a poor country, antenatal care should be provided before radiotherapy for cancer)	Make the best use of resources in providing interventions deemed worthwhile (for example, have nurses as opposed to doctors provide most antenatal care)	Equal access for equal need (for example, equal waiting time for treatment for patents with similar conditions)	Unequal treatment for unequal needs (for example, unequal treatment of those with trivial versus serious conditions)

Source: Mills and Ransom (2001).

An alternative approach to describing health care systems

Another way of describing a health system is based on the concept of *root definitions* (Checkland 1981) which suggests that any system involving human activity can be defined by six elements. These can be remembered by the mnemonic CATWOE:

- *Customers:* beneficiaries or victims affected by the system's activities
- *Actors:* those who carry out, or cause to carry out, the system's activities
- *Transformation process:* the means by which defined inputs are transformed into defined outputs
- *Weltanschauung:* the vision of the world assumed for the system to function; it makes the particular system a meaningful one to consider
- *Ownership:* a person or an agency having a prime concern for the system and the ultimate power to modify or to demolish it

- *Environment:* the constraints of the system in its environment (geography, national wealth) and in related or wider systems (educational, legal and financial).

Weltanschauung is a concept associated with the German sociologist Karl Mann-heim, meaning a comprehensive *world view*, from a particular standpoint. Think, for example, of the changing *Weltanschauung* in the sixteenth century when people shifted from believing that the earth was the centre of our universe to believing it was the sun. The term includes general assumptions as to the meaning of life, how things work and what is important. Obviously there is more than one possible world view related to health systems. An example is the extent to which concern for health should be based on altruism or self-responsibility. Remember also the importance of national culture as a determinant of health care, as discussed in Chapter 3.

Ownership is a complex concept, which not only relates to property rights but also has a cultural dimension; for example, the sense of ownership required to make community participation work. Think also of the example from the previous chapter of staff developing a sense of ownership for quality assurance. The import-ant question is who has the ultimate power to modify a system, for example to close a health centre, or to make a project fail.

A 'root definition' of a system provides a succinct description based on each of the CATWOE elements. It enables you to state in one sentence what the system is. For example, academic education is a publicly controlled system which, under observance of entry requirements, rewards students with academic degrees, subject to passing examinations held by teachers, who share the belief that advancement should be based on achievement.

 Activity 13.3

You probably had no difficulty in identifying the CATWOE elements in the above root definition. Think now of a health care system you are familiar with and construct a root definition using the CATWOE elements.

 Feedback

Obviously the *Weltanschauung* element varies with cultural context, and also between people acting in the system. So you need to find out the prevailing world view relevant to the system. For example, a root definition could describe the British NHS as:

A system for meeting the health needs of the entire population (transformation, customers) through the activities of those working in the National Health Service (actors, implied ownership by government), within limited resources (environ-mental constraints) and in the belief that health care free at the point of delivery is a good thing and most health professionals are essentially altruistic (*Weltanschauung*).

Summary

Comparison of health systems needs to be made in a meaningful way. Given the complexity and plurality of health systems it is difficult to obtain generalizable results. Various methods have been developed, including ideal types, multidimensional models and systems analysis. In this chapter you have seen how a systems approach provides a conceptual framework to define health systems using the CATWOE elements.

References

Checkland P (1981) *Systems Thinking, Systems Practice*. Chichester: Wiley.

Donaldson C, Gerard K (1993) *Economics of Health Care Financing: The Visible Hand*. Basingstoke: Macmillan.

Kohn R, White KL (eds) (1976) *Health Care: An International Study*. London: Oxford University Press.

Mills AJ, Ransom K (2001) The design of health systems, in MH Merson, RE Black, AJ Mills (eds) *International Public Health, Diseases, Programs, Systems, and Policies*. Gaithersburg, MD: Aspen.

OECD (1992) Sub-systems of financing and delivery of health care, in OECD, *The reform of health care*. Paris: OECD.

Roemer MI (1991) *National Health Systems of the World (Vol 1: The Countries)*. Oxford: Oxford University Press.

WHO (1999) *The World Health Report 1999: Making a Difference*. Geneva: WHO.

Why are health systems as they are?

Overview

In the previous chapter you learned about the different approaches to analysing health systems. In this chapter you will explore why health systems are as they are. You will consider the different theories which have been put forward to explain health systems and look more closely at the role of the state in health care.

Learning objectives

After working through this chapter, you will be better able to:

- **describe the role of state intervention in health systems**
- **outline the theories explaining the evolution of health systems**
- **give examples of factors influencing the convergence and divergence of health systems.**

Key terms

Convergence/divergence Processes, influenced by different factors, promoting similarities/ dissimilarities between health systems.

Corporatism Interest representation through professional organizations.

Sickness (sick) funds Non-governmental purchasing organizations in social insurance schemes.

The role of the state

A key issue in the formation of theory on health systems is the role of the state. What responsibility does government take for health services? Does the extent of state intervention vary between different health systems? If so, why? And what are the options for government intervention in the health sector?

 Activity 14.1

To understand better these questions think of the following scenario. Suppose a government has obtained a report that homeless people receive no appropriate health care. What are the basic options for the government in dealing with this problem?

Feedback

Your answers should include the following options.

1 Do nothing, ignore the problem.

2 Delegate the problem to other groups in society. Set rules or incentives for charities or the private sector to pay attention to these patients. In this option government takes the role of regulator.

3 Provide government-funded services for this group. The government acts as a funder; services may also be provided by the government or purchased from non-governmental organizations.

Obviously each option reflects a differing level of responsibility that government is prepared to take in this particular issue. In this example, reference is to the micro level of a specific programme. You may similarly look at the macro level of the health system and compare the types of state intervention in different countries. As the next activity shows, this helps to understand current trends underlying the development of health systems and helps to build a theory of state intervention in health care.

Classifying health care systems

The following extract from an article by Julio Frenk and Avedis Donabedian (1987) describes one approach to classifying national health care systems. They focus on two aspects (or 'modalities' as they call them): the form of state control and the basis of people's eligibility to use the system. (Remember, this was written in the 1980s, since when some significant changes have occurred in some of the countries cited.)

 Activity 14.2

While reading, think of the health system of a country you are familiar with and assess where it would fit in the matrix. Also consider the following questions:

1 What factors might be used to classify state intervention?
2 What factors are proposed to define the extent of state control?
3 How is eligibility categorized?

 State intervention in medical care: types, trends and variables

Defining modalities

Modalities are defined on the basis of one or more relevant attributes; the precise specification of these attributes becomes the crucial conceptual problem in defining the modalities and, hence, in developing a classification scheme. The choice of classifying attributes remains a controversial point in the literature on comparative health systems . . .

At least part of the disagreement may be due to the fact that the number of possible characteristics that could be used to classify state intervention in medical care is fairly large. . . . potential criteria for classification include the forms of payment to providers, the degree of administrative centralization, the number of public agencies involved in medical care, the means employed by the state apparatus to control the provision of services, the extent of coverage of the population, the number and kinds of benefits to which the covered population is entitled, and the basis for determining eligibility.

It is clear that no typology can incorporate all dimensions, since the large number of resulting categories would make the classification meaningless. A choice of criteria, even if arbitrary, has to be made. The element of arbitrariness can be reduced, however, if the criteria are selected using a theoretical framework which the typology is meant to serve. Accordingly, we have used as a guide Johnson's (1972) conceptualization of professional work, particularly the notion that state intervention represents a form of mediation between the producers and the consumers of medical services. The result is a typology based on two fundamental dimensions. The first, *the form of state control over the production of medical services*, reflects the relationship of the state to the providers of services. The second, *the basis for eligibility*, indicates the relationship of the state to the actual or potential consumers. Table 14.1 presents the resulting classification of modalities of state intervention in medical care.

Form of state control: relationship to producers

With respect to the first dimension, it is necessary to distinguish state control from simple public regulation. Furthermore, there are different forms and degrees of state control. Sometimes the state limits its role to the financing of care, while providers act essentially as private contractors. At other times the state may assume the direct ownership of health care facilities, with individual practitioners working as state employees. In the former case, the government is simply a buyer in the medical care market; in the latter, it is a producer. Other things being equal, ownership means a higher degree of state control than financing alone.

It is also necessary to take account of the administrative structure through which the state either buys or produces medical care. In any given organization, administrative control can be measured by several indicators. For our present purposes, however, it is enough to indicate the overall degree of control that the state can exercise through each intervention modality. To do so, we distinguish those modalities where state control is *concentrated* in a single agency or programme from those where control is *dispersed* among several agencies. The distinction is important because concentrated modalities signify greater state control than dispersed ones. There is, of course, a whole gradient of intermediate situations between these two extremes, but we have chosen to simplify the classification by focusing on the basic division between concentrated and dispersed administrative expressions of state control.

We have also adopted certain rules for classification. For example, whenever a federal health care programme is administered by state or province-level organizations in a modular fashion that allows for constrained variation, we judged the situation to be an instance of concentrated state control. In contrast, the presence of more than one independent agency, with substantial variation in administrative procedures and benefit levels, we classified as dispersed control, even when a central organization regulates or coordinates the agencies. Note also that the category of dispersed control includes cases where there are multiple agencies *within* a modality. The typical example is a social insurance scheme administered by several sickness funds.

Table 14.1 Typology of modalities of state intervention in medical care, with illustrative examples of each type

Form of state control	Basis for eligibility		
	1. Citizenship	2. Contribution/privilege	3. Poverty
A. Concentrated ownership	**A1.** National health service in most socialist countries; most of the national health system in Sweden; hospital care in the British National Health Service; hospital care in the national health insurance schemes of New Zealand and several Western European countries	**A2.** Social security in Spain; social security in Venezuela; social security in India; health care for the military in many countries	**A3.** Public assistance in many non-socialist underdeveloped countries
B. Dispersed ownership	**B1.**	**B2.** Social security in Mexico; public ownership sector of the USA federal government (Veterans Administration, Indian Health Service)	**B3.** Public assistance in many non-socialist underdeveloped countries; state and municipal hospitals and clinics in the USA
C. Concentrated financing	**C1.** National health insurance in Canada, New Zealand (ambulatory care), France (ambulatory care and part of hospital care); general practice in British National Health Service	**C2.** Social security in Brazil; social security in Lebanon	**C3.** Medicaid in the USA
D. Dispersed financing	**D1.** National health insurance in the Federal Republic of Germany, Austria, Switzerland, Belgium, Japan; catastrophic public medical insurance in the Netherlands	**D2.** Social security in Argentina: non-catastrophic public medical insurance in the Netherlands; public medical insurance sector in the USA (Medicare, CHAMPUS, Federal Employees Health Benefits Program, Workers Compensation)	**D3.**

Source: Frenk and Donabedian (1987).

The combination of the two expressions of state control (ownership plus financing or financing only) with the two administrative arrangements (concentrated or dispersed control) yields the four categories of the first dimension of our typology, which are shown as the row tabs in Table 14.1.

The basis for eligibility: relationship to consumers

With respect to the second dimension of the typology, it is possible to identify three principles for establishing which groups in the population are eligible for medical services that are either financed or directly provided by the state . . . (1) citizenship, (2) contribution/privilege and (3) poverty. Under modern definitions of citizenship, eligibility based on the first principle includes all or nearly all the population. Indeed, this principle derives from the notion that medical care is a social right not dependent on financial contribution, previous service to the state or indigence. There is, nevertheless, an important difference between potential eligibility and actual population coverage. In the process of ascertaining whether or not a modality belongs to the category of eligibility based on citizenship, it would be necessary to go beyond official declarations and include the extent of actual coverage. One would need some criterion, say the inclusion of 85 or 90 per cent of the population, that would make it possible to accommodate those situations where a modality approaches universality but does not quite cover 100 per cent of the population.

In contrast to citizenship, the remaining two principles of eligibility are selective; they do not include all the population. Beyond this similarity, there are fundamental conceptual differences between the two principles. In one case, the state can finance or provide medical services to particular subgroups of the population because they have contributed directly to that end (as in selective insurance schemes) and/or not because they have been made the privileged beneficiaries of state action (armed forces, civil servants, or certain workers perceived to occupy strategic positions in society). On the other hand, when the basis for eligibility is poverty, the state provides or finances medical services, not as a matter of privilege, but as a form of assistance precisely to the least privileged groups of a society. Consequently, the establishment of financial need becomes a necessary, though often not sufficient, condition for eligibility.

. . . The utility of this typology, and some of its other characteristics, can be appreciated by examining the illustrative selection of cases provided in the table. Besides its obvious ability to classify modalities of state intervention at any given time, the proposed typology can reveal certain worldwide patterns. We see, for example, that not all modalities are equally likely in practice. So far, we have found no cases of state intervention characterized by dispersed ownership and by eligibility based on citizenship (cell B1). This absence shows that the dimensions of the typology are interdependent. It would seem, for example, that the political, ideological and economic conditions that allow a state to undertake the direct provision of services to the whole population are hostile to the fragmentation of control among multiple agencies.

Two other very infrequent modalities are those by which the state limits its role to that of only financing medical services to the poor. In one of them (D3) there seem to be no cases, and in the other (C3) the only current case is represented, to the best of our knowledge, by Medicaid in the United States. Such a scarcity of cases may reflect the fact that, by trying to subsidize the assimilation of the poor into the mainstream of private medicine, these modalities go against the long-standing practice of providing medical services to the poor through a separate state-owned system.

Apart from those modalities that, traditionally, were not used, or only rarely used, there are others that are now relatively infrequent but which in the past were much more often encountered. For example, purchasing services for limited population groups on the grounds of contribution or privilege (cells C2 and D2) used to be much more common than it is now, at least in Europe. The earliest social insurance programmes in Europe could be placed in these segments of our typology, since they were directed only to wage earners earning less than a specified level of income and generally excluded their dependants as well as the self-employed, the peasantry and the middle and upper classes (Starr 1982) . . .

Another important feature of our approach is that an entire nation can be characterized on the basis of which and how many modalities exist within it and their relative importance. In this way cross-national comparisons of the extent and nature of variation in state intervention can be made. The procedure of classification and comparison can be carried out for finer political subdivisions within a nation.

 Feedback

1 Frenk and Donabedian suggest seven possible defining characteristics: forms of payment to providers; degree of administrative centralization; number of public agencies involved in care; means used by state to control provision; extent of population coverage; number and kinds of benefits for entitled population; basis for determining eligibility.

2 Two factors are used to define state control: whether or not the state's role extends beyond financing to include direct ownership of services; and how centralized or dispersed the state's administrative control is.

3 Eligibility is categorized as: citizenship (universal); based on people's financial contributions or privileges; and based on socioeconomic status (i.e. poverty).

Why do health systems evolve?

Examining the historical context can contribute to understanding how health services have evolved over time. For example, analysing the development of industrial relations explains how different interest groups of employers and trade unions have shaped the evolution of health services. However, the political standpoints from which historical processes are seen differ and have given rise to at least three theories.

Popular choice

The *popular choice theory* assumes that health systems have developed as they are, because the *public wants* the system it has. According to Ginzberg (1992): 'It is still the citizen who through their voice in the marketplace and in the legislature determines how their money will be allocated.' Popular choice has been used to explain, for example, why the USA relies more on private than on public health services.

Power groups

Obviously the popular choice theory underestimates the influence of actors within the health services and so it has been complemented by other writers such as Starr (1978) who have analysed the influence of *power groups* on the health system. In their view the system is a function of the different degree of power that the health care professions, hospitals, insurance companies and the drugs and supplies industry have in the decision making process (similar to the discussion of environmental turbulence in Chapter 2).

Marxist theory

The *Marxist approach* is associated with writers such as Navarro (1986) and Elling (1980) who argue that health systems have been shaped by the power relations between social classes. National health programmes have mainly been established by the influence of the labour movement, through its trade unions and political parties. International differences in health systems can be understood by analysing the degree to which class aims have been achieved. This depends on the relative strength of the industrial working class in relation to the capitalist class, and its ability to forge alliances with other classes, such as farmers.

 Activity 14.3

1   How does the health system in your country differ today from the way it was 100 years ago? You may need to find out more about the way it used to be.
2   Consider the extent to which each of the three evolutionary theories explains the changes that have occurred.

 Feedback

1 You should have considered changes in such aspects as financing, ownership, extent of separation of purchasing from provision, role of the state, power of the health care professions and eligibility for services.

2 You probably found that each of the three theories explains some aspects of the changes that have occurred but that none of them can account for all the changes. This is a fairly common finding and simply shows that no one theory can satisfactorily explain all phenomena.

How have health systems evolved?

Do health systems become more similar over time or not? This is the question of *convergence* or *divergence*. Proponents of convergence have argued that demographic changes and increasing wealth of nations have led to common solutions in the health sector. Health systems are converging in ensuring more equitable and better health services. But is that true? Critics have pointed at the widening gap between low and high income countries and interpreted the destabilization of health systems in low income countries as a sign of divergence. No doubt the debate is politicized, with proponents of convergence theories being associated with the political right and divergence theories being associated with their Marxist critics.

 Activity 14.4

The following is another extract from the paper by Frenk and Donabedian (1987) that considers the arguments as to whether systems are converging or diverging. As you read it, consider which factors influence divergence and convergence of health systems. Give one example of each from the text or from previous chapters.

 Are systems converging or diverging?

Convergence: a world-system approach

Industrialization and urbanization

The process of development almost everywhere in the world is accompanied by large-scale economic and political changes that include the increasing dependence of workers on labour markets and wages, the concentration of manufacturing in factories, the growth of cities, the spread of political mobilization and the consolidation of state power. There is widespread agreement on the crucial role played by some of these changes, especially those linked to industrialization and urbanization (Mechanic 1975), in stimulating the intervention of nation states in medical care. This effect is seen most clearly in the growth of social insurance and social security systems worldwide. As Sigerist (1943) asserted, 'social insurance is a result of the industrialization of the world' . . .

Part of this convergence is attributable to the dynamics of industrialization and urbanization as they unfold within any given society. For instance, the dependence on a labour market for cash income, which has accompanied the advance of industrialization and wage work, has caused insecurity among industrial workers everywhere. In addition, industrialization has contributed to state intervention by sharpening the need to maintain a healthy labour force capable of achieving the high levels of productivity required by industrial enterprise.

Industrialization not only creates the need for protecting the working population against the risks of sickness and disability, but also provides the means of attaining that protection. Thus, the spread of wage work and the concentration of workers in urban factories create the resources and opportunities for financing special sickness funds and for developing an organized network of medical care facilities. A similarity across nations in both the needs created and the opportunities offered by industrialization seems to account for at least part of the trend toward convergent modalities of state intervention in medical care.

In terms of the two dimensions underlying the proposed paths to state intervention, the advance of industrialization has had a direct impact on the extension of coverage as larger segments of the population have been incorporated into the industrial system of production. And, as indicated earlier, to the extent that industrialization paves the way to roughly similar methods of financing and organizing medical care, it also tends, other things being equal, to produce convergence in the degree of direct state control over the production of medical services.

The medical world economy

As Mechanic (1975) points out, there is an 'international knowledge, technology and manpower marketplace' in the field of medicine. It is beyond the scope of this paper to analyse the determinants and dynamics of the various sectors of that marketplace, which include the diffusion of knowledge through meetings, journals and textbooks, the transfer of technology through multinational pharmaceutical and medical equipment companies and the migration of medical personnel facilitated by the standardization of training programmes. Each of these sectors tends to create, throughout the world, the conditions for a model of medical work based on complex organizations that, in most cases, can only be financed and operated by the state. Even in the face of very dissimilar patterns of disease, practically every nation state accepts and implements scientific medicine and the high-technology practice that derives from it. Almost everywhere, hospitals have become the central organizations for the provision of care, and physicians with fairly equivalent training have become the dominant practitioners. In the vast markets created by a medical world economy, the state has increasingly been called upon to take the lead as the only actor with enough resources to be an effective buyer, or with sufficient power to control the other powerful actors in the international private sector . . .

The world ideology of modernity

The world ideology of modernity has been a major factor leading to convergence among countries and the provision of services by a complex state apparatus has become a characteristic of advanced and underdeveloped societies alike. A health care system has become part of the institutions of modernity, and the participation of the state in such a system has become part of the definition of a modern nation state. The world ideology of modernization and progress has made it legitimate for states to be actively involved in the organization, financing and delivery of health services to their own peoples, and to collaborate with other nations on efforts explicitly pertinent to health.

Some of the most important components of the world polity are international organizations. These organizations have transcended their initial concerns with the negative impact of epidemics on commercial and military expansion. Nowadays, international bodies cover every aspect of health care organization and have been prominent in the diffusion of the paradigm of scientific medicine . . .

Two sets of considerations have contributed to the legitimacy of state intervention in medical care. The first is the acceptance of health care as a right. This principle, which is an extension of the concepts of civil and political rights to the realm of social affairs, can be expected, as it is more widely implemented, to produce cross-national convergence toward greater population coverage on the grounds of citizenship alone.

The second set of considerations arises from an expansion in the legitimate functions of medicine. Modern medicine provides systems of explanation and strategies for action which are presented as rational alternatives to folk or moralistic interpretations of experience. Indeed, medical explanations and solutions have expanded beyond the phenomena of disease, strictly defined, to encompass an increasing set of objects, ranging from certifying physical and mental normality to verifying the quality of air, water and housing; from crime and drug abuse to child rearing, sexuality and the full array of human habits.

Divergence: internal variables

It is not infrequent to find expressions of amazement about the great similarities among the health care systems of countries that differ vastly in economic development and socio-political organization. Actually, the contrary is equally amazing. Given all the forces for convergence discussed above, it is truly remarkable that individual nation states continue to exhibit such a wide range of variation in the levels and forms of state intervention in medical care. As we have seen, these differences are not random; they have patterns that the profiles of modalities and the paths to state intervention we proposed attempt to capture. What is needed next is a set of variables that can account for these persistent dissimilarities. As indicated earlier, such variables operate within each nation state. They include economic factors (namely, the structure of the medical care market), political forces (the system of interest representation) and ideological definitions (i.e. norms about the legitimacy of auspices and ownership).

Structure of the medical care market

The structural characteristics of the market for medical services immediately before a governmental health programme is introduced seem to limit the range of options available to that programme. As a consequence, differences in the structure of the medical care market among countries are a source of corresponding dissimilarities, or divergence, in their forms of state intervention, even though state intervention itself may subsequently alter the market structure in fundamental ways . . .

System of interest representation

Since the nineteenth century and, even more so, since the end of the Second World War, medical care has become an object of political demands, collective bargaining, partisan programmes and group pressures. The forms of health care delivery that have emerged from the interplay of these forces have been shaped by the institutional arrangements that the organized groups of civil society use to negotiate their interests with the state. Because these arrangements differ from country to country, their main effect has been a contribution to divergence among the modalities and paths of state intervention in medical care.

From among the many industrial arrangements that represent partisan interests, the one most relevant to our analysis is the extent of corporatist representation of the various occupational groups engaged in the production of medical services, most especially of physicians. We use the term 'corporatism' in a broad sense, to refer to a system of interest representation characterized by hierarchical and non-competitive occupational associations, which represent their members' interests through direct negotiations with the state (Schmitter and Lehmbruch 1979) . . .

Norms about legitimacy of auspices and ownership

. . . Differences among countries as to who may legitimately own, operate or employ the resources required to produce medical care are likely to be reflected in differences in the modalities of state intervention in health care, particularly in the degree of direct state control. A radical redefinition in the norms governing auspices and ownership seems to have been a very important element in the rapid increase of state control among socialist countries . . . Even within modality A1 (Table 14.1), a major difference between the socialist countries, on the one hand, and nations like England and Sweden, on the other, lies in the fact that the latter have preserved a legitimate arena for private practice. Moreover, as described during the earlier discussion of backward movements along a path, a redefinition of the norms of ownership and auspices can sometimes occur in the direction of reduced state control. Another example of how these norms can produce persistent differences among nations is provided by the United States. The fact that Medicaid represents, to the best of our knowledge, the only large-scale government programme that purchases health care for the poor, rather than providing it directly, may be related, at least in part, to strong ideological commitment to the private enterprise system in the United States.

 Feedback

Factors for convergence include:

- *industrialization and urbanization* – for example, 'social insurance is a result of industrialization of the world' (Sigerist 1943);
- *the medical world economy* – 'International knowledge, technology and manpower marketplace' (Mechanic 1975);
- *the ideology of modernity* – seeing health care as a right, protected by the modern nation state; expansion of modern medicine to other areas of social life.

Factors for divergence include:

- *structure of the medical care market* – availability of private care in the health sector of a country at the time of change;
- *system of interest representation* – corporatist or non-corporatist representation of physicians in relation to interest representation of other groups in society;
- *norms about legitimacy of auspices and ownership* – for example, strong commitment to private ownership in the USA, leading to reduced state control over the health sector.

Summary

In this chapter you have looked at different theories explaining why health systems have developed as they have and examined the role of state intervention in this process. Control of ownership and finance and the basis of eligibility of users for access to publicly funded services are important dimensions explaining differences between health systems. Various factors have been suggested to influence convergence and divergence in the form of state intervention in health care.

References

Elling RH (1980) *Cross-national Study of Health Systems: Political Economics and Health Care*. New Brunswick, NJ: Transaction Books.

Frenk J, Donabedian A (1987) State intervention in medical care: types, trends and variables. *Health Policy & Planning* 2: 17–31.

Ginzberg E (1992) *The Medical Triangle: Physicians, Politicians and the Public*. Cambridge, MA: Harvard University Press.

Johnson TJ (1972) *Professions and Power*. London: Macmillan.

Mechanic D (1975) The comparative study of health care delivery systems. *Annual Review of Sociology* 1: 43–65.

Navarro V (1986) *Crisis, Health and Medicine: A Social Critique*. New York: Tavistock Publications.

Schmitter PC, Lehmbruch G (eds) (1979) *Trends towards Corporatist Intermediation*. Beverly Hills, CA and London: Sage.

Sigerist HE (1943) From Bismark to Beveridge: developments and trends in social security legislation. *Bulletin of the History of Medicine* 8: 365–88.

Starr P (1978) Medicine and the waning of professional sovereignty. *Daedalus Journal of the American Academy of Arts and Science* 107: 175–93.

Starr P (1982) *The Social Transformation of American Medicine*. New York: Basic Books.

15 Low and middle income countries: from colonial inheritance to primary care

Overview

In the previous two chapters you explored the different approaches to studying health systems, looked more closely at the role of the state and discussed some of the trends in health care which are similar in low, middle and high income countries. In this and the following two chapters you will examine the salient differences between low/middle and high income countries, looking first at the organization of health services in the former, from the colonial era to the present day, and then at some important trends in health services in high income countries.

This chapter begins with an overview of the history of health services in low and middle income countries and an explanation of the concept of primary care. You will learn that each of the primary care principles needs an appropriate approach to planning and management of health services. You will also focus on the debate on comprehensive versus selective primary care.

Learning objectives

After working through this chapter, you will be better able to:

- give examples of factors shaping health services in low and middle income countries
- outline the principles of primary care
- describe obstacles to the implementation of the Alma-Ata approach to primary care
- conceptualize the approach of selective primary care.

Key terms

Burden of disease A measure of the physical, emotional, social and financial impact that a particular disease has on the health and functioning of the population.

Comprehensive primary care A comprehensive health strategy (outlined in the Alma-Ata Declaration) based on equity, a multisectoral approach, community participation, appropriate technologies, and health promotion.

Decentralization The transfer of authority and responsibility from central government to local levels, which are thereby strengthened.

Horizontal programmes Health services organized to provide care across a range of diseases at one level (usually primary care).

Selective primary care An interim strategy until comprehensive primary care is available for all, based on selection of cost-effective medical interventions.

Vertical programmes Health services focused on a single disease or population group (such as children) encompassing all levels of care.

Influences on health services in low and middle income countries

In this book you have seen many differences between low, middle and high income countries. At this stage you are going to explore these differences more systematically. The following activity will help you to understand why it is important to do so.

 Activity 15.1

Write notes on how economic, political, sociodemographic, geographic and historical factors influence health services organization in low and middle income countries.

 Feedback

You probably thought of many factors. Here are some examples:

Economic factors:

- lower national income, meaning lower spending levels on health care and greater scarcity of resources (discussed in Chapter 7);
- unequal distribution of wealth between the few rich people and the majority of the population living in poverty;
- travel costs to health services being an obstacle to achieving equity.

Political factors:

- instability with frequent changes of government;
- displaced populations – There are approximately 50 million refugees worldwide, the majority in low income countries;
- external influences (e.g. World Bank) encouraging contraction of the state and cuts in publicly funded programmes;
- self-determination movements (women, farmers, trade unions) fighting for civil liberties and participation in health care issues.

Sociodemographic factors:

- large differences in population density causing logistic problems for health services;
- difficulties in providing facilities and attracting staff to remote areas;
- high growth rates of the population, leading to increasing demand for health care;
- rapid urbanization, meaning floating populations and disintegration of traditional structures;
- unequal access to education (particularly for girls) resulting in high illiteracy levels;

- epidemiological transition from communicable to non-communicable diseases (see Table 15.1).

Geographical factors:

- prevalence of 'tropical' diseases;
- natural conditions and catastrophes influencing agriculture, communication, transport and nutritional status.

Historical factors:

- colonial inheritance;
- concentration of facilities in urban areas;
- centralized planning;
- imbalances between curative and preventive services.

Table 15.1 Epidemiological transition

Groups of disease	High income countries 2000	Low income countries 2000	Low income countries 2020
1. Communicable nutritional pregnancy-related	8%	33%	19%
2. Non-communicable	84%	53%	64%
3. Injuries and violence	8%	14%	17%

Source: Murray and Lopez (1996).

The colonial inheritance

Health services organization in many low income countries has been shaped by their colonial past which explains many of the present-day differences between countries (Abel-Smith 1986). For example:

- in British colonies, services were provided mainly for the army and civil services and later extended to the indigenous population
- in French colonies, government services were less developed and mainly based on larger employers who were responsible for providing health services
- in Spanish colonies there was a tradition of government and charity hospitals with the introduction of social insurance schemes in the twentieth century.

It is notable that health systems development has been different in countries that were never colonized; in these countries there has been a greater role for private sector provision. After gaining independence, most countries extended existing services to more of the population as far as available resources allowed. In this process, missionary health services played a role. Emphasis was put on good basic care and community outreach programmes. In addition, countries started their own training programmes for health care workers.

International initiatives to promote primary care

Low and middle income countries responded to the problems in different ways. The introduction in China in 1957 of 'barefoot doctors' brought about a reorientation of health services towards primary care. Similar models of primary care were developed in Kerala (southern India) and Sri Lanka. The Arusha Declaration in 1967 led to a shift in health policy in African countries. Its aims included a radical change in the development philosophy and replacement of the colonial administration with trained nationals. Based on a framework of socialism and self-reliance, the declaration stressed participatory decision making, an equitable income distribution and rural development.

Villages were emphasized as the appropriate units of cooperative production. Programmes to increase the literacy rate, the availability of clean water, immunization rates and access to mother and child health care were designed and often successfully implemented (Jonsson 1986).

The 1978 Alma-Ata Declaration can be seen as a result of the changing trends towards primary care that were part of the thinking about organization of care in the previous decade. The Alma-Ata Declaration was important in bundling these convergent trends and formulating a consistent strategy to achieve health care for all. The key themes and philosophy of the Declaration were described by Andrew Green (1999).

The Alma-Ata Declaration

The broadening of the concept of health, an understanding of the wider causes of ill health, a desire to incorporate a greater involvement of communities in decision-making, a shift in developmental thinking towards social ends, and a recognition of the inappropriateness of many of the health-care structures inherited by developing countries to tackling their predominant health problems. These themes formed the backdrop to the 1978 Alma-Ata Conference ... The resultant declaration endorsed primary health care (PHC) as the means of attaining the WHO goal of Health For All.

The Declaration is important on at least two levels. Firstly, it expresses a philosophy of thinking about health and health-care. Thus, running through it are five themes. These are:

- the importance of equity as a component of health
- the need for community participation in decision-making
- the need for a multisectoral approach to health problems
- the need to ensure the adoption and use of appropriate technology
- an emphasis on health-promotional activities.

In addition, since Alma-Ata, two further themes have emerged, which were implicit within the Declaration. They are decentralization and the involvement of a variety of health sector agencies (as distinct from other sectors such as education). The principles of PHC are universal, in that they are considered relevant for any country at any point in time ... At a second level the declaration listed particular essential service interventions. These are:

- education concerning prevailing health problems and the methods of prevention and control
- promotion of food supply and proper nutrition
- adequate supply of safe water and basic sanitation
- maternal and child health-care, including family planning
- immunization against the major infectious diseases

- prevention and control of locally endemic diseases
- appropriate treatment of common diseases and injuries
- provision of essential drugs.

All of these elements are again universal basic requirements, although many higher-income countries have already attained basic levels. As a result the Alma-Ata Declaration was for a long time, unfortunately, associated primarily with the needs of developing countries.

The declaration was perhaps also unfortunate in its choice of the term 'primary health care'. This term already had connotations. It had been used in many countries such as the UK to refer to the first level of care. As a result, the spirit of the Declaration regarding the principles referred to above has been applied in some instances to primary care *services* alone. Both the principles of appropriateness of technology and equity imply the need for the development of such an infrastructure of basic services. However, this is a limited interpretation of PHC without reference to the whole of the health system, other sectors, or the need to involve communities in decision-making.

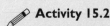 **Activity 15.2**

Green went on to identify potential obstacles to implementation of the approach advocated by the Declaration. As you read the following edited extract, note the main obstacles to implementation that concerned him.

 Obstacles to implementing the Alma-Ata Declaration

Twenty years after the adoption of the Alma-Ata Declaration, many countries still have not fully internalized the philosophy in such a way that it is reflected in their planning systems and strategies. Various different reasons can be put forward to explain why the early optimism, following Alma-Ata, has not always been justified.

Misinterpretation of the PHC concept

It has already been suggested that the philosophy of PHC has been misunderstood by some. This has led to emphasis on the primary level of care, or to particular components of the strategy, such as community health workers, frequently called PHC workers, to the exclusion and neglect of other parts of the health system. Other misinterpretations centre around the principles of community participation, with undue emphasis being given to resourcing and community financing rather than empowerment.

Selective PHC strategies

A second reason for the failure to adopt the PHC philosophy fully can be traced to suggestions that it was not feasible in the short term with the resources available. An alternative to what became known as *comprehensive PHC* was promoted, and became known as *selective* PHC. The strategy of selective PHC suggests that priority diseases be chosen for intervention, based on centrally predetermined criteria. This has resulted, in some countries, in vertical disease-led approaches which run counter to the idea (central to PHC) of integrating services. The use of centrally determined criteria for the selection of these health problems also reduces the possibility of community involvement in setting priorities. It also implies a return to a medical model of health, and ignores the importance of development in its widest sense. Lastly, at a practical level, it fails to recognize the importance of building up an adequate infrastructure from which particular programmes can be built . . .

Resistance to change

The third and most significant factor which has constrained the development of PHC is the resistance encountered from a variety of groups. Various groups have felt (rightly in some cases) threatened by the philosophy of PHC. Some health professionals have been concerned at the erosion of their power. Commercial interests, such as the drug industry, have been concerned at a potential loss of markets.

More fundamental, however, is political resistance. Some politicians have seen the emphasis on social justice, equity, participation, and empowerment as challenging existing political structures and their own position within them. PHC has been described as a revolutionary philosophy and, indeed, if taken to its logical conclusion, it would require a complete change in the political structure and situation of a number of countries. The principles of PHC have far greater significance than to the delivery of health services alone. The broader concept of health that we have outlined, and which includes social justice, is immensely challenging to the political structures of many countries . . .

Centralized management and planning infrastructure

Lastly, the failure of some countries to implement PHC policies can be attributed in part to the failure of the planning and management infrastructure. Attention in a number of countries in recent years has focused on policies to decentralize health management decision-making structures. Such policies, as we have seen, may stem from the principles of community participation and multisectoralism. In recent years increasing attention has been paid to decentralization as part of wider interest in health system structures.

 Feedback

The main obstacles identified by Green were:

1 misinterpretations of the concept

2 lack of resources, leading to technocratic solutions of 'selected' primary care

3 political resistance – emphasis on social justice, empowerment and participation seen as a challenge to politicians

4 centralized management and planning.

 Activity 15.3

This activity requires you to draw on what you have read, while thinking in practical terms about the implementation of primary care in your country. The differences in approach to primary care in low, middle and high income countries are explored in the feedback.

The questionnaire below is designed to help you draft a profile of primary care in your country.

Primary health care in *(name of country)*:

1. Describe the approach to PHC

2. Does PHC reflect the following principles? (Answer yes or no and give brief reasons for your answer.)

   • Equity

   • Community participation

   • Multisectoral approach

   • Appropriate technology

   • Emphasis on health promotion

3. List the professions that are members of the PHC team

 Feedback

Compare the information you gave with the following discussion.

The five principles (equity, community participation, the multisectoral approach, appropriate technology and emphasis on health promotion) are universal principles of any primary care system. But many countries have never implemented this approach systematically. There is a large gap between rhetoric and the reality of primary care.

Though the organization of care varies considerably in high income countries, the following staff are often included in primary care: doctors (generalists), nurses, social workers, health visitors, midwives, counsellors, physiotherapists and occupational therapists.

In low income countries, where there are fewer doctors, community health workers (CHWs) are the first point of contact with the health system for most people. Teams may include paramedics, birth attendants, nurses, midwives, health inspectors and family planning officers.

The selective–comprehensive primary care debate

Primary care following the Alma-Ata Declaration led to an expansion of services and increased managerial complexity. Huge progress was made with vertical programmes which focused either on one disease, such as TB, or on one patient group, such as children. These contributed to reducing mortality. However, many programmes failed to address the intersectoral issues, that is, problems that required the input of sectors other than health such as education or housing. Primary care became an agenda only for health services. Community participation became rhetorical or focused only on mobilization of funds rather than on participation in decision making. The experience with CHWs was mixed, with the WHO (2000) reporting the failure of some schemes.

Community health workers

Over the past twenty years many countries have experimented with the use of community health workers (CHWs) to provide primary health care. Several African countries introduced CHW programs in the 1970s as a way of extending primary health care services at low cost nationwide. Health workers' responsibilities typically include providing education on sanitation, nutrition, family planning, child health, and immunizations, in addition to carrying out some basic health interventions. They can also be valuable as a referral point between health centers and the community. Regrettably, CHW programs have had mixed results. Studies have shown that in the Gambia and Indonesia traditional birth attendants who were not backed up by skilled services were unable to decrease the risk of maternal mortality.

A Jamaican program, launched in 1977, that used CHWs in primary health care efforts is an example of a well-intentioned effort gone awry. Problems emerged from the beginning, with the selection of personnel. CHWs generally demonstrate greater dedication when they serve the communities in which they live. Unfortunately, too few CHWs were recruited from the target communities, and workers who lived elsewhere had to be enlisted. Inability to recruit male volunteers limited the success of family planning and STD-prevention programs. The CHWs – a large group – sought and obtained civil service benefits, including a set salary structure and promotion opportunities. In 1985 salaries for briefly trained CHWs were to be equivalent to two thirds those of registered nurses with three years' training. Health center buildings were altered to serve as bases for CHW operations. Shortages of higher-level staff prompted many health centers to substitute CHWs for nurses, even though the workers lacked the necessary training. CHWs became increasingly linked to the health system, but their availability to the community diminished. The program has since been greatly reduced.

Other efforts have been more successful. Perhaps the largest scale NGO-run community health worker program is the Pastoral da Criança, operated by the Catholic Church in Brazil. This program, initiated in 1983, receives strong support from the Ministry of Health and some technical and financial support from UNICEF and from the Bernard Van Leer Foundation and other NGOs. It now has 47,000 CHWs throughout Brazil. An estimated 1.5 million children were enrolled in the program in 1992. CHWs provide health education to low-income mothers regarding the importance of prenatal care, good diet during pregnancy, breastfeeding, proper weaning, immunizations, and management of diarrhea, and they monitor the growth of infants and young children. The training process for CHWs follows a central guideline but is adapted to fit the characteristics of different regions. Special care is given to the training programs for illiterate volunteers, and supervision of CHWs is closely integrated with continuing education and motivational support. An evaluation carried out in 1990 found that health and nutritional indicators for young children enrolled in the program were significantly better than indicators from similar communities in which the Pastoral da Criança had no activities.

Community health workers are also central to the successful Aga Khan Health Service primary health care programs in remote mountainous areas of rural Pakistan. The CHWs – volunteers selected by the villagers – collect epidemiological information, provide health education, identify problems, and provide simple treatment and referrals. They are backed up by mobile teams of physicians and nurses.

The assumption that comprehensive primary care was appropriate and affordable was re-evaluated during the 1980s. The main argument for a shift in policy was the finance problems. It was recognized increasingly that primary care for all was not cheap and that logistic and organizational problems had been underestimated. The expectations that increasing resources would be available for primary care failed. On the contrary, the economic crisis in the 1980s forced governments to cut back public expenditure.

This shift in policy led to the emergence of the concept of selective primary care. An understanding of the debate between proponents of comprehensive and select- ive primary care is important for three reasons:

- It will show you how decision making can be based on economic evaluation of interventions. This gives you a better understanding of subsequent policies based on the essential packages of care approach in low income countries.
- The critics of a selective approach give a perspective which is often missed by managers who focus only on the success of their particular programme.
- The debate is important too for middle and high income countries. It exempli- fies the dilemmas of priority setting in health care.

The following describes the approach Julia Walsh and Kenneth Warren proposed in 1980 for selecting health care interventions. Don't worry about the medical details – the emphasis is on the method. The authors argue that until comprehensive primary care is made available to all, a selective approach 'may be the most effect- ive means of improving the health of the greatest number of people'. This is called a burden-of-disease approach to priority setting.

Selective primary health care: an interim strategy for disease control in developing countries

In selecting the health problems that should receive the highest priority for prevention and treatment, the following factors should be assessed for each disease:

- prevalence
- morbidity or severity of disability
- risk of mortality
- feasibility of control (including relative efficacy and cost of intervention).

It cannot be overemphasized that the greatest immediate efforts in health care in less developed areas should be aimed at preventing and managing those few diseases that cause the greatest mortality and morbidity and for which there are medical interventions of relatively high efficacy. As a demonstration of a typical approach to selective health care we might arrive at Table 15.2, incorporating the four factors listed above.

Table 15.2 represents the beginnings of a cost effectiveness analysis of typical illnesses that all may be endemic in a less developed nation or area. All may present threats to public health, but it may not be possible to control all three infections simultaneously on a large scale. The importance of taking into account feasibility and cost of control as well as mortality and prevalence is made clear in Table 15.2. The newly discovered Lassa fever carries a 30–66% mortality in the few limited outbreaks seen in Nigeria, Liberia and Sierra Leone. Those who survive recover fully after an illness of 7–21 days. Its high fatality rate would seem to give it high priority for a major health program. However, its mode of transmission is not known, and its treatment is difficult: injections of plasma from recovered patients are required. Because no attempts have been made to develop a

Table 15.2 Comparison of potential opportunities to control three infectious diseases

Infection	Prevalence	Mortality	Morbidity	Feasibility of control
Lassa fever	Unknown: thought to be low	High (30–66%)	Moderate (bedridden 7–21 days)	Extremely poor at present
Ascariasis	Extremely high: thought to affect 1 billion people	Extremely low (approximately 0.001%)	Low (minor disability and often asymptomatic)	Fair (long-term to indefinite drug treatment required)
Malaria	High: more than 300 million infected annually	Low (approximately 0.1%)	High (severe, many complications, often recurrent)	Good (chemoprophyiaxis available: regular spraying programs for vectors practical)

Source: Walsh and Warren (1980).

vaccine, Lassa fever is impossible to control at present. Therefore, concentration on preventing Lassa fever would not do the greatest good for the greatest population. Ascariasis or roundworm is the most prevalent infection of man, infecting one billion people throughout the world. Its human burden is enormous and no one can deny the importance of alleviating it. Yet, fortunately, disability is minor and death from ascariasis is infrequent. Treatment requires periodic chemotherapy administered indefinitely. Control may ultimately require massive, long-term improvements in sanitary and agricultural practices in order to reduce the inevitability of continuous reinfection. The difficulty of eliminating exposure to the roundworm as well as the low intensity of the infection would lead us to rank ascariasis as deserving less attention than its ubiquity would seem to require.

Malaria has a far smaller mortality rate than Lassa fever in terms of virulence, and a lower prevalence than ascariasis. Yet its mode of transmission is well known and it produces much recurring illness and death – about 1 million children in Africa alone die from malaria. It is endemic to Africa, Central and South America, and the Caribbean, the Indian sub-continent and Eastern Asia, and travellers frequently carry it elsewhere. What also distinguishes malaria from Lassa fever and ascariasis is that it frequently can be effectively and relatively inexpensively controlled through regular mosquito spraying programs or chemo-prophylaxis. Of these three infections, then, assigning malaria the highest priority for concentrated prevention and control would be the most effective way to reduce overall morbidity and mortality.

Using the process outlined above for Lassa fever, ascariasis and malaria, we evaluated the major infections endemic to the developing world and assigned high (I), medium (II), or low (III) priorities. Within categories exact rank is not of major significance and it may change depending on the geographic area under consideration. Furthermore, even the priorities themselves may have to be modified depending on the climate and flora and fauna of a particular area. For instance, schistosomiasis, to which we assigned a high priority, is restricted in distribution and the infection may not be a significant health problem in all areas of the world. Our results and rationale for the proposed hierarchy are listed as Table 15.3.

Table 15.3 Priorities for disease control based on prevalence, mortality, morbidity and feasibility of control

Infection	Reasons for assignment to this category
I. *High*	
Diarrheal diseases	High prevalence, high mortality, high morbidity, effective
Measles	control
Malaria	
Whooping cough	
Schistosomiasis	
Neonatal tetanus	
II. *Medium*	
Respiratory infections	High prevalence, high mortality, no effective control
Poliomyelitis	High prevalence, low mortality, effective control
Tuberculosis	High prevalence, high mortality, control difficult
Onchocerciasis	High morbidity, medium prevalence, low mortality, control difficult
Meningitis	Medium prevalence, high mortality, control difficult
Typhoid	Medium prevalence, high mortality, control difficult
Hookworm	High prevalence, low mortality, control difficult
Malnutrition	High prevalence, high morbidity, control complex
III. *Low*	
South American trypanosomiasis (Chagas disease)	Control difficult
African trypanosomiasis	Low prevalence, control difficult
Leprosy	Control difficult
Ascariasis	Low mortality, low morbidity, control difficult
Diphtheria	Low mortality, low morbidity
Amebiasis	Control difficult
Leishmaniasis	Control difficult
Giardiasis	Control difficult
Filariasis	Control difficult
Dengue	Control difficult

Source: Walsh and Warren (1980).

Group I represents the infections causing the greatest amount of most easily preventable illness and death: diarrheal diseases, malaria, measles, whooping cough, schistosomiasis, and neonatal tetanus. With the exception of schistosomiasis, all the infections receiving highest priority for health care planning affect young children more than adults. Together with respiratory infections and malnutrition, they account for most of the morbidity and mortality among infants and young children . . .

Groups II and III encompass health problems of lesser importance or less amenability to containment. Again, feasibility of control in light of limited resources is an influential factor in the analysis. Respiratory infections, a major cause of disability and death, are not listed in Group I because of difficulties in their prevention and management . . .

We assigned a disease a medium or low priority if we found a lack of inexpensive control measures for it. For example, there is no therapy for chronic Chagas disease. Only toxic drugs and procedures of unknown efficacy, such as nodulectomy, are available for treatment for onchocerciasis. Leprosy and tuberculosis require years of drug therapy and even longer follow-up periods to ensure cure. Rather than attempting immediate large-scale treatment programs for these infections, the most efficient use of resources may be investments made in research and development of less costly and more efficacious means of prevention and therapy.

 Activity 15.4

Choosing a country that you are familiar with, find out how resources are distributed between the major areas of need (diseases or population groups). You will need to consult sources of national statistics. Then consider to what extent the distribution is based on the burden-of-disease criteria proposed by Walsh and Warren. Finally, consider the reasons for any mismatch.

 Feedback

You will probably find there is some (but only some) correspondence between burden of disease and service provision. The reasons for any mismatch are likely to be predominantly political and historical.

Summary

The colonial era has left low income countries with a legacy of centralized and unequally distributed health services. Primary care is a strategy of reorienting health services according to the principles of equity, community participation, intersectoral interventions, appropriate technology and health promotion. Each of these principles needs to be addressed by appropriate management activities. Lack of resources, political resistance and misinterpretations of the concept are among the reasons for failure to fully adopt the approach and are still obstacles to its implementation. A response to these problems is the strategy of selective primary care – you have examined the positions of advocates and critics of this concept.

References

Abel-Smith B (1986) Global perspective on health service financing. *Social Science & Medicine* 21: 957–63.

Green A (1999) *An Introduction to Health Planning in Developing Countries* (2nd edn). Oxford: Oxford University Press.

Jonsson V (1986) Ideological framework and health development in Tanzania 1961–2000. *Social Science & Medicine* 22: 745–53.

Murray C, Lopez A (1996) *The Global Burden of Disease. Vol. 1*. Geneva: WHO.

Walsh JA, Warren KS (1980) Selective primary health care: an interim strategy for disease control in developing countries. *Social Science & Medicine* 14C: 145–63.

WHO (2000) *World Health Report*. Geneva: WHO.

16 Low and middle income countries: from comprehensive primary care to global initiatives

Overview

In the previous chapter you saw how health services in low and middle income countries developed from the colonial era to the 1980s. You also examined the debate on selective and comprehensive primary care. In this chapter you will review important initiatives in low and middle income countries, which have shaped the organization of health services from the 1980s to the present. This chapter gives you an opportunity to explore in particular the policy of an essential package of care, the Bamako Initiative, the reforms that have been implemented in low income countries under the auspices of the World Bank, and the more recent sector-wide approaches and global initiatives.

Learning objectives

After working through this chapter, you will be better able to:

- **describe the essential package of care approach**
- **outline the main international initiatives intended to reorganize health services in low income countries**
- **conceptualize the changing roles of state and private sector in health services finance and provision.**

Key terms

Bamako Initiative An international initiative in 1987 based on PHC principles with focus on community financing and decentralization.

Community financing Collective action of local communities to finance health services through pooling out-of-pocket payments and ensuring services are accountable to the community.

Disability-adjusted life years (DALYs) A measure of health based not only on the length of a person's life but also on their level of ability (or disability).

Essential package of care A strategy for purchasing services that achieves the greatest reduction in the burden of disease with available resources.

The essential package and the district model

As you saw in the previous chapter, many governments faced the fact that comprehensive primary care was more expensive than expected. The economic crisis in the 1980s gave rise to a further departure from the comprehensive concept. The increasing debt burden and structural adjustment programmes often led to cuts in essential primary care. Many of these reforms were inspired by and directed under the auspices of the World Bank which took over the leading policy role in low income countries from the WHO.

Among the important ideas in the early 1990s was the *package* concept put forward by the World Bank. It was seen as a way to maximize community effectiveness of interventions and it was a compromise on the selective-comprehensive debate, as the new policy acknowledged the importance of the supportive services and intersectoral policies. The model has the following inputs:

- *essential health care* – immunization, ante- and postnatal care, maternal services, family planning, and basic outpatient care
- *supporting services* – information, education and communication to improve screening and diagnostic accuracy, provider and patient compliance
- *intersectoral interventions* – safe water supply and sanitation.

As you can see, the approach again emphasizes intersectoral interventions. The following activity requires you to reflect on the importance of this issue.

Activity 16.1

Look at Figure 16.1. What does the relationship between female literacy and health status of children suggest for planning of health services in low income countries?

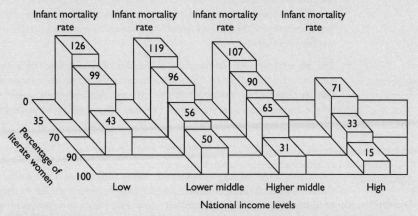

Figure 16.1 Infant mortality and women's literacy, by broad income group (Ellencweig 1992)

Feedback

> Investment in education (particularly for females) and measures that strengthen the status and rights of women are central to a health strategy. The example also shows the importance of combined maternal and child health programmes, which can be used for information and education on health issues. As you can see, major determinants of health are to be found outside the health sector.

The Bamako Initiative

Another important shift in policy was related to the Bamako Initiative, a declaration following the meeting of African ministers of health in 1987. The declaration restated the principles of primary care with a strong focus on decentralization.

 Activity 16.2

> The following short account by Barbara McPake (1994) explains what the Bamako Initiative was and gives examples of how community co-finance works. What interpretation of community participation underlies the initiative?

 Initiative for change

The Bamako Initiative . . . aimed to revitalise the public sector health care system, involving the community in decisions about local health services and strengthening district management. It proposed that new approaches to financing local health services – such as user fees, pre-payment schemes or revolving drug funds – be introduced to generate funds that would be fed back into improving or extending local health services. By 1993, thousands of health centres in 30 countries (including three non-African countries) were participating in the Bamako Initiative.

The term 'community co-financing' is broader than 'user fees' because it emphasises the community's role in determining what reforms should be introduced and in managing, as well as contributing, resources. It also stresses that financial support from higher levels of the health system is important. The key difference between the two approaches is community accountability through their involvement in decision-making.

Studies have shown that when user fees for health services are centrally planned and imposed, people are less likely to use health facilities and the income raised is small. Experience in Africa suggests that community co-financing is more effective than user fees. Evidence from the two West African countries of Benin and Guinea showed increased use of health facilities (although from very low levels) and the potential for generating income, which could be kept for use at the local level.

The main way of involving communities is through a health management committee at each health facility level. Committees can be directly or indirectly elected by the community, formed from other existing committees, such as development committees, or older committees can be reformed. Deciding how community co-financing will be implemented is often the reason for setting up a committee. Committees later undertake wide-ranging responsibilities. These include how to use funds, monitoring, management of finances, and considering wider community needs.

Health management committees can give communities a stronger voice in decisions about local health services, and are a way to ensure that health workers are accountable to communities. In Guinea, committees refused to pay bonuses to city health centres with more staff than was necessary.

One problem is ensuring that communities are truly represented on a committee. For example, in Rwanda in central Africa some committees were dominated by their chairmen, included few women and were not well known among the communities they should have represented. Much is expected of committees. Research by UNICEF shows there are 29 separate tasks that the committees must undertake. It is unlikely that any community committee is tackling all these tasks successfully.

An evaluation of Bamako Initiative activities in five African countries in 1992 suggested that the range of tasks and the limited management skills of committees may restrict the degree of community involvement in decision-making that is possible. The evaluation stressed the importance of identifying and strengthening ways by which communities could be supported rather than undermined.

The lessons from current experience suggest that to bring about community participation in decision-making requires monitoring, supervision, appropriate training and the development of management tools for use by the community. Directing community participation to a number of key tasks, as done in some countries such as Guinea and Rwanda, seems to allow effective support and effective involvement.

 Feedback

A key component of the Bamako Initiative was participation of communities in managing and financing health services. It was mainly seen as a way to mobilize additional resources for the health sector. This interpretation does not necessarily imply that communities have a voice in decision making.

Remember the range of possible interpretations of the term 'community participation': it can be seen as a strategy of empowerment or simply as a means to raise money for health services, which were formerly free. This shows once again how the discourse on a subject can be used to express different interests.

Community finance spread to countries in other continents, involving a variety of schemes, such as revolving drug funds (in which a community pays the drugs supplier after it has sold them on to patients) and rural health insurance. There is evidence that community co-financing can improve utilization and quality of services, if funds are kept at the local level (Levy Bruhl et al. 1997).

Agenda for Reform and World Development Report

In 1987 the World Bank published an *Agenda for Reform* (Akin 1987) which advocated the introduction of user fees in low income countries and a long term policy for the introduction of health insurance. This set the health policy agenda for the late 1980s. It took up the theme of a smaller role for government in health care but emphasized a more centralized approach to finance than the Bamako Initiative. It is important to understand that this initiative was influential in redefining the roles of the public and private sector in health care. As a consequence it led to massive changes in finance and provision of health services in low income countries.

The *World Development Report* (WDR), which was published by the World Bank in 1993, incorporated the earlier ideas of user fees, health insurance and decentralization. The concept of the essential package of care was taken further to an essential public health package and an essential clinical package. Importantly, the report also advocated a redefinition of the roles of states and markets in finance and provision of health services.

The essential features of the WDR can be summarized as:

- financing – with an emphasis on user fees and insurance
- structural change – decentralization, with an emphasis on the district and local level
- redefinition of the role of the state – government to focus only on essential services, encourage private sector finance and provision of health services.

The following is an overview of the key messages and the agenda for action of the WDR report. Note that the report uses a more comprehensive measure to assess the burden of disease than Walsh and Warren (Chapter 15); it is based on the number of disability-adjusted life years (DALYs) lost from premature death, injury and disease. Similarly, the cost-effectiveness analysis is based on DALYs gained per dollars spent.

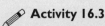 **Activity 16.3**

Compare the three-pronged approach to government policies adopted by the report with the selective primary care approach that you read about in Chapter 15.

 Investing in health: key messages from the WDR 1993

Foster an environment that enables households to improve health

Household decisions shape health, but these decisions are constrained by the income and education of household members. In addition to promoting overall economic growth, governments can help to improve those decisions if they:

- Pursue economic growth policies that will benefit the poor (including, where necessary, adjustment policies that preserve cost-effective health expenditures)
- Expand investment in schooling, particularly for girls
- Promote the rights and status of women through political and economic empowerment and legal protection against abuse.

Improve government spending on health

The challenge for most governments is to concentrate resources on compensating for market failures and efficiently financing services that will particularly benefit the poor. Several directions for policy respond to this challenge:

- Reduce government expenditures on tertiary facilities, specialist training, and interventions that provide little health gain for the money spent.
- Finance and implement a package of public health interventions to deal with the substantial externalities surrounding infectious disease control, prevention of AIDS, environmental pollution, and behaviors (such as drunk driving) that put others at risk.
- Finance and ensure delivery of a package of essential clinical services. The comprehensiveness and composition of such a package can only be defined by each country, taking into account epidemiological conditions, local preferences, and income. In most countries public finance, or publicly mandated finance, of the essential clinical package would provide a politically acceptable mechanism for distributing both welfare improvements and a productive asset – better health – to the poor.
- Improve management of government health services through such measures as decentralization of administrative and budgetary authority and contracting out of services.

Promote diversity and competition

Government finance of public health and of a nationally defined package of essential clinical services would leave the remaining clinical services to be financed privately or by social insurance within the context of a policy framework established by the government. Governments can promote diversity and competition in provision of health services and insurance by adopting policies that:

- Encourage social or private insurance (with regulatory incentives for equitable access and cost containment) for clinical services outside the essential package.
- Encourage suppliers (both public and private) to compete both to deliver clinical services and to provide inputs, such as drugs, to publicly and privately financed health services. Domestic suppliers should not be protected from international competition.
- Generate and disseminate information on provider performance, on essential equipment and drugs, on the costs and effectiveness of interventions, and on the accreditation status of institutions and providers.

Increased scientific knowledge has accounted for much of the dramatic improvement in health that has occurred in this century – by providing information that forms the basis of household and government action and by underpinning the development of preventive, curative, and diagnostic technologies. Investment in continued scientific advance will amplify the effectiveness of each element of the three-pronged approach proposed in this Report. Because the fruits of science benefit all countries, internationally collaborative efforts, of which there are several excellent examples, will often be the right way to proceed.

 Feedback

The approach taken in the WDR is broader and a more plural strategy for health development. It also puts emphasis on intersectoral activities, for example economic growth, poverty relief, female education and rights and status of women.

In contrast, selective primary care is a narrow strategy focusing only on health care interventions. The idea of selecting interventions is taken further by the WDR, as it adopts the approach of the essential package of health services. Unlike the selective primary care approach, the WDR uses a more sophisticated method to assess burden of disease, which includes measures of disability.

The changing public–private mix

The policies of the WDR were influential in shaping the organization of health services in low income countries. Most countries introduced user fees and many have adopted the essential package of health care approach.

This goes along with a contraction of the state in finance and provision of services. Many countries have reduced government activity and promoted private health care, often without sufficient evidence of the quality and efficiency of the services provided by private providers. Governments have devised policies to regulate the private sector. However, a major problem is to monitor compliance and enforce rules. Country examples of radical privatization include China where, with the breakdown of the commune system, services were extensively privatized, and Chile, where steps to privatization were taken by the Pinochet regime in the early 1980s (Bennet *et al.* 1997).

Sector-wide approaches

The importance and relevance of intersectoral work was taken forward in the 1990s with sector-wide approaches (SWAps), programmes agreed between the governments of low income countries and bilateral donors (Cassels and Janovsky 1998). Such agreements were based on:

- a collaborative programme of work in line with agreed policies
- the establishment of management systems, especially around financial management
- expenditure plans
- putting funds into a common pool or basket to support the programme of work.

Global health initiatives

The involvement of both public and private finance to support health services was extended to the contribution of donors as the new century dawned (Brugha *et al.* 2002). These global public–private partnerships involved the input not only of well-established international bodies such as WHO but also of philanthropical organizations (such as the Bill and Melinda Gates Foundation) and pharmaceutical companies. Given the source of such support, it is not surprising that there is considerable interest in the provision of new drugs and vaccines. These initiatives largely focus on particular diseases (HIV, TB, malaria) or on vaccination and immunization programmes. As such they adopt a vertical approach. They aim to:

- improve access to sustainable immunization services
- expand the use of all existing safe and cost-effective vaccines and promote delivery of other appropriate interventions
- support the national and international accelerated disease control targets for vaccine-preventable diseases
- accelerate the development and introduction of new vaccines and technologies

- accelerate research and development efforts for vaccines needed primarily in developing countries
- make immunization coverage a centrepiece in international development efforts.

In a review of progress over the first 18 months in four sub-Saharan countries, Brugha *et al.* (2002) found that while the initiative was welcomed, the pace of implementation was too rapid. Problems included low staffing levels in districts, insufficient transport and fuel, poorly functioning cold chains (to maintain the viability of vaccines) and infrequent supervision. There was also concern that the high cost of new vaccines would be difficult to sustain if funding by the Global Alliance for Vaccines and Immunization (GAVI) ended after the initial five year commitment.

 Activity 16.4

These findings have relevance for a subsequent public–private initiative, the Global Fund to fight Aids, Tuberculosis and Malaria (GFATM). These concerns are expressed by Peter Poore (2004) in the following edited article. As you read it, note what his main worries are.

 The Global Fund to fight Aids, Tuberculosis and Malaria

Most diseases can be controlled. With adequate investment, short-term success can almost always be guaranteed in any setting. In the poorest countries, however, such success will be limited unless the more fundamental causes of poverty and inequity are also addressed. This requires that the world's poorest be freed from the cycle of debt, unfair trade restrictions and undemocratic international policymaking that protects the wealthy at the expense of the poor.

The Global Fund (GF) was created in 2002 in response to growing international concerns about the global impact of these diseases. It is a new financial instrument, not an implementing agency . . . To date it has disbursed over US$113 million to programmes in 53 countries and committed $1.5 billion over 2 years to 154 programmes in 93 countries.

In the lowest income countries, there have been many attempts over the last few decades to galvanize political commitment and financial support for the control of specific diseases . . . Few if any have had continued success beyond that commitment and that financial support, either because it was not sustained or was insufficient to reach all of those in need.

The GF is a new financial instrument with innovative approaches to project approval and the management of resources. But let us be clear about the real problem that the GF is addressing. Firstly, it is not a technical problem . . . Secondly, it is not a financial problem . . . The real problem lies in a culture of self-interest where international aid and investment is designed in the interests of the donor, and where the donors' conditions take precedence over the recipients' needs.

Despite billions of dollars having being spent in aid over the last few decades, it has been insufficient to the needs of the poorest countries, insensitively invested and frequently inappropriate to local context. As a result, it has also been largely ineffective in reducing poverty in these countries . . .

However, money alone is not enough. Of greater importance is finding ways to spend it in the interests of the recipient, according to their needs and in line with their capacity to absorb these additional funds over time . . . Failure to sustain investment hit precisely those countries that were least able to afford continuing costs. In response to these limitations, many donors and governments moved to support longer-term investment through sector-wide approaches. Such an approach focuses on establishing and maintaining effective systems of delivery, including the recruitment of properly trained and supported staff, common to all diseases . . .

The GF seeks donations from all sources, including the traditional donors, in theory without the limits and conditions imposed by individual governments and institutions. It can disburse those funds indefinitely, provided it can continue to attract funds, and become the first initiative that is truly 'financially sustainable'. However, as with other initiatives, it expects others to take-up the 'challenge of future financing'. So, the GF is new, but how will it be different? . . .

Two features are common to many disease-specific campaigns. The first is that most claim that whilst reducing disease, they act as 'catalysts' to attract continuing support for successful interventions. A laudable aim, but too often in the past large projects designed in the wealthy countries have been 'kick started' with large international grants, with little attention to local contexts, only to leave the recipients to pick up the recurring bills when the initial investment runs out. The second is that they claim that they will 'spearhead' the development of comprehensive health care systems on the back of successful disease control and in the process contribute to economic development and poverty alleviation. There is very little evidence of this having happened in the poorest countries up to now (UNDP 2003).

. . . Although there is no doubt that many people will benefit from the GF, it seems likely that it will face the same limitations of all short-term project-based attempts to address the fundamental problems underlying the prevalence of these and other poverty-related diseases in the poorest countries . . . There is a risk that well funded projects can distort the more comprehensive provision of care by attracting staff and other resources to the project area. They can also distort government efforts at planning for long-term solutions to national health care needs. If the GF aims to ensure that investment remains adequate over time and is also sufficient to reach all of those in need for as long as is necessary, then it must establish a monitoring process that reflects this aim. Relevant indicators that go beyond recording funds disbursed and the number of diseases avoided will be crucial.

Feedback

Poore has a number of concerns, including: the need to address the fundamental causes of poverty and inequity; the difficulties of sustaining any benefits if the Global Fund is short term; the motivation and aims of donors who may be acting out of self-interest; and technical obstacles to implementation in impoverished communities.

Activity 16.5

An alternative, and more optimistic view, is put forward by Vinand Nantulya (2004), a senior advisor to the Global Fund, in which he argues that this initiative differs from previous ones in key aspects. As you read the following, note the four ways the Global Fund is thought to differ.

 ### The Global Fund: what makes it different

The Global Fund is about shifting the present paradigm. First, it is demand-driven. Countries develop and submit proposals to the GF that provide creative solutions to critical gaps in their existing national strategies: solutions that integrate responses to HIV/AIDS, tuberculosis and malaria with poverty reduction; and solutions that aim to strengthen the health infrastructure and human resource capacity to ensure sustainability.

Secondly, the GF is an inclusive partnership, reflected at country level by the idea of a country coordination mechanism (CCM). The role of CCMs is to bring together government, non-governmental organizations (NGOs), faith-based organizations, bilateral and multilateral technical agencies, academia, the private sector, labour, the media, and people living with these conditions . . .

Thirdly, the disbursement of funds to countries is to be performance-based, linking financial accountability to programme performance. The different interests within the CCMs should make it possible for performance to be measured in a transparent and accountable manner. Furthermore, Local Fund Agents, appointed by the GF to serve as its ears and eyes on the ground, will monitor and verify country processes . . .

Fourthly, the GF underlines the need to coordinate donor input at country level, regardless of source, to achieve synergy. Existing national coordination structures and systems, such as the National AIDS Councils, Roll Back Malaria, and Stop TB partnerships, should be enhanced by the umbrella forums provided by the CCMs.

In conclusion, a paradigm shift is possible. But strengthening the health systems, developing human resource capacity, addressing poverty, and achieving outcome and impact level results will take time. Moreover, resources through the GF should be additional to, and not a substitution for, existing allocations . . . and recipient countries should be exploring innovative ways for scaling up existing activities and addressing absorptive capacity issues.

 Feedback

Nantulya suggests that the Global Fund is

1 demand (recipient country) driven

2 an inclusive partnership of relevant stakeholders

3 performance-based

4 coordinated with activities of other donors.

Summary

The economic recession in the 1980s exacerbated the financial problems of health services and led to a policy shift from comprehensive primary care to priority setting through measures of burden of disease and intervention effectiveness. A number of international activities were influential in changing the financing and provision of health care. The reforms in the 1990s were related to searching for new financing methods and structural changes. They go along with a redefinition of the roles of the state and the market in health care, leading to reduced government activity and a greater role for the private sector. Since 2000, there has been renewed interest in vertical programmes through global health initiatives funded from a combination of public and private sources.

References

Akin JS (1987) *Financing Health Services in Developing Countries: An Agenda for Reform*, World Bank policy study 0258–2120. Washington, DC: World Bank.

Bennet S, McPake B and Mills A (eds) (1997) *Private Health Providers in Developing Countries: Serving the Public Interest?* London: Zed Books.

Brugha R, Starling M, Walt G (2002) GAVI, the first steps: lessons for the Global Fund. *Lancet* 359: 435–8.

Cassells A, Janovsky K (1998) Better health in developing countries: are sector-wide approaches the way of the future? *Lancet* 352: 1777–9.

Ellencweig AY (1992) Health systems – a critical analysis of existing and suggested models, in AY Ellencweig, *Analysing Health Systems, A Modular Approach*. Oxford: Oxford University Press.

Levy Bruhl DL, Soucat A, Osseni R *et al.* (1997) The Bamako Initiative in Benin and Guinea: improving the effectiveness of primary health care. *International Journal of Health Planning and Management* 12(Suppl. 1): 49–79.

McPake B (1994) Initiative for change. *Health Action 9* (June–August): 7.

Nantulya VM (2004) The Gobal Fund to fight AIDs, Tuberculosis and Malaria: what makes it different. *Health Policy & Planning* 19: 54–6.

Poore P (2004) The Global Fund to fight Aids, Tuberculosis and Malaria (GFATM). *Health Policy & Planning* 19: 52–3.

UNDP (2003) *Human Development Report 2003*. New York: United Nations Development Programme.

World Bank (1993) *Investing in Health: World Development Report, 1993*. Washington, DC: World Bank.

17 Health services in high income countries

Overview

In the previous two chapters you explored the organization of health care in low and middle income countries. In this chapter you will look at some trends in the way the delivery of health care in high income countries is currently changing. The chapter gives you an opportunity to revise some of the concepts you have come across in this book and looks more closely at the interrelationships between different levels and forms of care, in particular at the concepts of referral and substitution between different forms of care.

Learning objectives

After working through this chapter, you will be better able to:

- describe substitution between different forms of care as a key instrument of health care reform
- give examples of different types of substitution and outline advantages and difficulties of implementation
- outline the changing role of hospital and primary care in high income countries.

Key terms

Appropriateness A health care intervention is deemed appropriate if the benefits that result outweigh the costs (all aspects, not just financial) by a sufficiently wide amount.

Intermediate care Residential or inpatient care for those who have been in hospital but are not yet ready to go home and for those who need inpatient care but are not so ill as to require the services of a major hospital.

Length of stay The length of time a patient stays in hospital.

Meta-analysis An overview of all the valid research evidence; if feasible, the quantitative results of different studies may be combined to obtain an overall result, referred to as a 'statistical meta-analysis'.

Skills mix The mix of posts, grades or occupations in an organization. It may also refer to the combinations of activities or skills needed for each job within the organization.

Substitution A process replacing existing services with more appropriate ones, through changes in location of care, technology, and staff and skills mix.

The changing patterns of care

In earlier chapters you have seen the importance of the appropriate use of different levels of care. In particular, primary care plays an important role in providing the first contact with health systems and, in some countries, acting as a gatekeeper to secondary and tertiary care. However, organizational patterns change over time. There is a continuous adaptation process between clinical practice and the organization of health services. Think, for example, of mentally ill people who used to be treated in hospitals and are now treated in the community: community care has *substituted* for hospital care. The process of substitution is a general phenomenon. It is helpful to distinguish between three kinds of substitution:

- Changing *location* – these are changes in the type of institution, for example giving birth at home instead of hospital.
- Introducing new, more effective *technologies* – such as TB chemotherapy, facilitating treatment in primary care instead of a sanatorium.
- Changing *mix of staff and skills* – substitution between different professions or changes in skills mix, such as nurse practitioners substituting for doctors or specialists in geriatric medicine replacing general physicians.

You need to be aware that the concept of substitution is related to appropriateness of care. For example, it is an important management strategy to reduce the number of inappropriate admissions to hospitals or to match services with the appropriate mix of skills and staff. Replacing an established form of care with a more appropriate one affects outcomes, for example increased patient satisfaction, and may involve lower costs.

 Activity 17.1

As you are probably aware, in most high income countries the number of hospital beds has declined. What factors have led to this?

 Feedback

Though there are still large international differences in the number of hospital beds per capita, the length of stay is getting shorter. This is due to more effective interventions, better coordination with primary care and better home conditions. For example, day case surgery and minimally invasive methods (e.g. keyhole surgery) have shortened the length of stay and the overall need for beds. More interventions are being performed as ambulatory (outpatient) care.

 Activity 17.2

The following is an extract from a review of research on skill mix by James Buchan and Mario Dal Poz (2002). It focuses largely on changes in roles between doctors and nurses and between nurses and health care assistants. As you read it, consider the following questions:

> 1 What are the three ways in which the relationship between two occupational groups can be altered?
> 2 To what extent can the research findings in one country be implemented in other countries?

 ## Skill mix in the health care workforce: reviewing the evidence

The *World Health Report 2000* (WHO 2000) noted that determining and achieving the 'right' mix of health personnel are major challenges for most health care organizations and health systems. Health care is labour-intensive and managers of health care provider units strive to identify the most effective mix of staff that can be achieved with the available resources, taking into consideration local priorities.

The term 'skill mix' is usually used to describe the mix of posts, grades or occupations in an organization (strictly speaking, this is more accurately referred to as 'grade mix'). It may also refer to the combinations of activities or skills needed for each job within the organization.

... There is no common starting point for examining skill mix in different countries, sectors and health systems. Resource availability, regulatory environments, culture, custom and practice will all have played a role in determining the typical or normal mix of staff in a particular health system. To the extent that these factors vary, so will the typical mix. Indeed there are marked variations between countries and regions in terms of the mix of health care occupations.

Use of existing professions

... The meta-analyses reviewed reveal evidence (mainly but not exclusively from the United States) that, in settings where there is actual or potential role overlap between registered nurses and doctors, there is scope for a cost-effective increase in the role and deployment of the former. In particular, the use of clinical nurse specialists, nurse practitioners and clinical nurse midwives can improve care outcomes (often measured by patient satisfaction), while maintaining or reducing costs.

... Substitution of cheaper care assistants for more expensive nurses for cost-containment purposes has become increasingly apparent in recent years in many countries. Many of the publications in this area are written by and for qualified nurses, and set out their concerns about being replaced or having their skills undervalued. These papers argue that a cheaper skill mix may be no more cost-effective because of the various hidden costs associated with skill dilution. This argument cites factors such as higher absence and turnover rates of less qualified staff; higher levels of unproductive time because care assistants have less autonomy and capacity to act independently; and reported concerns about possible harm to patients if care assistants are required to work beyond their technical or legislated capacity. Most of these studies tend to be unit-level before-and-after examinations of the effects of introducing or increasing the use of care assistants. There is no unanimity in results or conclusions, even setting aside issues of methodology and comparability.

... The model in use can be determined on the basis of whether the support staff are being used to supplement, complement or replace (substitute for) qualified nurses. Studies of the impact of the introduction of unlicensed assistants in the USA have shown mixed results.

Some have suggested a positive impact: cost savings using patient care assistants, and using nurse aides with no adverse effect on patient satisfaction. Other studies have been less clear cut, or have found the opposite, highlighting problem areas such as decreased quality and increased on-call work, sick leave and overtime working, reported higher workload for registered nurses and, initially, a higher turnover of patient care technicians, and a larger proportion of more highly qualified nurses being related to higher reported quality of care.

. . . Occupations other than nurses have received relatively little attention. In some countries, especially in Latin America and the Caribbean, there has been some examination of different mixes of technicians. Although the number of these technicians is large and growing in some cases, no analytical study was found. Studies on pharmacists tend to focus on an analysis of activity related to the control of prescriptions and expenditures or even on the interaction with patients and their families. Few studies attempt to evaluate the pharmacists' work in relation to that of other health workers.

Introductions of new types of worker

Many health systems have considered or implemented the introduction of new cadres or groups of health workers to fill a skills gap or improve the cost-effectiveness of the skill mix in the health workforce. In practice, these are often persons in existing occupations or grades with additional skills or an extended role. In some countries, such cadres have been most evident in rural and remote areas, where it may be difficult to recruit conventional health professionals. They include:

- conventional support workers (in catering, patient transport, cleaning, catering and food distribution, and clerical areas) who are multiskilled or have an extended role;
- care assistants and auxiliaries who are multiskilled, have undergone 'cross-training' or have an extended role (e.g. health community agents in the family health programme in Brazil);
- current health care professionals (e.g. nurse practitioners) with an extended role;
- technicians with new roles (e.g. in surgery or anaesthesiology, as in Mozambique).

The extent to which truly 'new' cadres of worker have been introduced to health systems is difficult to determine as there is much blurring of roles, with conventional workers being given extended roles, perhaps with a new job title. So are there new types of workers or simply new types of work being undertaken by existing staff? Moreover, cultural, professional and organizational differences mean that the role of a specified worker or professional in one country or health system may be different from that in another. Some country health systems have developed roles that are country-specific or system-specific, such as nurse anaesthetists, respiratory therapists and medical assistants/clinical officers in Africa; and physician assistants in the USA. Many of these roles have been developed as a solution for the shortage of doctors.

Conclusions

There are significant limitations to the current evidence on skill mix in the health workforce. Many published studies in this area are merely descriptive accounts, which add little in terms of use of methods or interpretation of results. Where studies do move beyond description, their usefulness is often constrained by methodological weaknesses, lack of appropriate evaluations of quality/outcome and cost, and/or use of small sample sizes. Moreover, many of the studies were undertaken in the USA, and the findings may not be relevant to other health systems and countries. The results may therefore be suspect, and of little use for comparative purposes or in drawing general conclusions.

... Despite these limitations ... the evidence suggests that increased use of less qualified (cheaper) nursing staff will not be effective in all situations, although greater use of care assistants has improved organizational efficiency. Evidence on the doctor/nurse overlap indicates that there is unrealized scope ... for extending the use of nursing staff and for further development of care delivery led by nurses/midwives, for example, in maternity units. The effectiveness of different skill mixes across other groups of health workers and the associated question of the development of new roles remain comparatively under-explored.

Feedback

1 The relationship between occupational groups may be changed by using one group to *supplement, complement or substitute for* another group.

2 Care must be taken in implementing research findings from one country in another country because the same benefits may not result in a different context. Context may differ in many ways: resources available, regulatory environment, culture, custom and history.

Primary care in high income countries

Though the Alma-Ata approach (see Chapter 15) is universal, there are large differences in the organization of primary care between high income countries. What all systems have in common is that primary care:

- is the first contact with the health system
- acts as gatekeeper to hospital care and to drugs
- to a varying extent, provides a multiprofessional approach to patients' needs.

The many differences in the organization of primary care between countries relate to:

- different forms of remuneration of providers, which have an impact on the utilization of services: the average number of consultations per week seems to be higher under a fee-for-service payment as compared to capitation or salaried payment
- different organizational arrangements – solo practices, group practices or multi-professional health centres and polyclinics
- different standards of training – requirements to practise as a doctor or a nurse vary widely
- differing extent of functional integration with community and social services
- access to specialist care varies from self-referral to only being able to gain access via a professional referral, usually a primary care doctor.

 ## Activity 17.3

Think of your country's health system and identify how primary care is organized, You will need to consider:

a) Service delivery
(solo practice/group practice/health centre/other)

b) Employment status of doctors
(independent contractors/employed/dual jobholding in joint private and public practice)

c) Population served
(geographically defined/list system/no defined population)

d) Prevailing remuneration of GPs
(salary/fee-for-service/capitation/other)

e) Referral restrictions
(gatekeeping/direct access to specialists)

f) Level of internal integration between staff
(uniprofessional; multiprofessional; teamwork)

g) Level of external integration with other services
(e.g. social services, public health, education services)

h) Level of integration of staff education and training in primary care
(undergraduate/basic; postgraduate/post-basic; continuous professional development)

Feedback

This activity should have helped you to identify how organizational issues affect the functioning of primary care. For example, highly fragmented health services pose problems of cooperation between different sectors (private, public, NGOs) or types of care (preventive, curative, rehabilitative). The type of facility affects integration of services; for example, health centres and group practices can offer more opportunities for multiprofessional work than solo practices. A key issue of strengthening primary care is appropriate training. Training of clinical staff has traditionally been hospital-oriented though is increasingly based partly in primary care.

Activity 17.4

Referring to Table 17.1, compare the distribution of the four professions shown between the 13 European countries included.

1 To what extent does the availability of each profession vary?
2 Which factors could explain the variation in the rate of provision of nurses between European countries?

Table 17.1 Health service inputs per 100,000 population for a selection of European countries (1995–2002)

Country	Acute care hospital beds	Physicians	Nurses	Dentists	Pharmacists
Albania	277	130	362	NA	NA
Austria	610	332	NA	NA	58
Czech Rep.	631	350	922	63	53
Finland	230	316	NA	NA	151
France	397	333	NA	NA	104
Germany	627	335	793	74	59
Italy	398	612	NA	NA	111
Lithuania	604	399	789	74	65
Netherlands	307	315	NA	NA	20
Slovakia	688	322	707	43	51
Sweden	228	304	NA	85	60
UK	241	NA	543	43	NA

NA = not available

Source: data extracted from WHO website.

 Feedback

1 Physicians vary in number by a factor of nearly 5, from 130 in Albania to 612 in Italy; nurses vary by a factor of 2.5, from 362 in Albania to 922 in Czech Republic; dentists vary by a factor of 2, from 43 in the UK and Slovakia to 85 in Sweden; and pharmacists by a factor of over 7, from 20 in the Netherlands to 151 in Finland.

2 Explanations for these variations could include:

- statistical factors (e.g. missing data)
- variations in definition of professions
- differences in roles of men and women, social status, income and working conditions.

Variations in definitions and the inconsistent application of internationally agreed definitions make these sorts of comparisons fraught with dangers (just as you saw for comparisons of funding in Chapter 7). The WHO definition of a nurse, for the purposes of these data is:

- completed basic nurse education of at least 2 years
- qualified and authorized to practise in own country
- working at least 35 hours a week.

For some countries but not others, the data on nursing numbers will include midwives, feldschers (physician assistants) and nurse specialists. Similar inconsistencies affect other measures, such as the number of beds, used to compare countries, so great care must be taken in interpreting any observed differences.

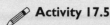

Activity 17.5

You will have seen in Table 17.1 another striking difference between countries – the availability of acute hospital beds. This varies from less than 250 per 100,000 population in Finland and the UK to over 600 in Austria, Czech Republic, Germany, Lithuania and Slovakia. This partly reflects historical differences but also recent changes in perceptions of the role of the hospital in modern health care. Many of the issues are raised by Nigel Edwards and Martin McKee (2002) in the following article. As you read it, consider two questions:

1   What are the factors that are leading to a reappraisal of the role of a hospital?
2   What changes to hospital functions do the authors suggest?

 ### The future role of the hospital

The hospital is perhaps the most enduring and visible symbol of a health care system. But what is a hospital for? Do the reasons why hospitals came into being and the principles that helped form them still apply? And what should a hospital look like in the future? These questions are especially relevant today as several countries embark on substantial programmes of investment in new facilities. It is unlikely that these new hospitals will last as long as some of their predecessors. But whatever decisions are made now will certainly have important consequences for how health care is provided for at least the next 30–50 years.

Although institutions described as hospitals have existed since the fourth century AD, the modern hospital had its origins around the beginning of the twentieth century. Developments in anaesthesia, control of infection and medical science and technology have created clinical and economic reasons for concentrating often scarce and expensive resources in purpose-built facilities. This incremental process has created a model that reflects its history but may be increasingly less appropriate for the future.

. . . The changes in medicine and increased specialisation that promoted the growth of hospitals are continuing and, together with restrictions in working hours, are greatly increasing the size of the population required to support a full range of services and provide a sufficient case load for clinicians to maintain their skills . . . The challenge is how to define a future role for hospitals that can deliver high-quality medicine but which also provides high levels of access to users and support to primary care and other services not based in hospital.

The answer to this question appears to lie in challenging whether the activities that currently take place in hospital really need to be there and whether the way in which services have been grouped together needs to continue.

[First], disaggregating the emergency services into different streams that recognise the needs of the patients rather than those of the provider creates a number of opportunities. The small numbers of patients with major trauma need a specialist service covering large populations supported by a wider trauma management system. However, over half of the users of hospital emergency services have conditions that can be treated by primary care and specialist minor injury services. Nurses and primary care doctors can provide this care locally without the support of hospitals. Removing these patients from the hospital also has a very positive impact on the remaining emergency services.

[Second], patients requiring assessment and diagnosis are more appropriately managed in a setting where the staff have time and facilities to undertake it rather than in a busy emergency room or accident department. Streamlined protocols combined with rapid investigation mean that the decision to admit or discharge can be made much more quickly. Many of these patients already go home very quickly and improving the assessment process offers further opportunities for this. Integrating these services into local disease management initiatives may offer even more scope for reducing the reliance on hospital-based care. If in future there are fewer hospitals, there will be a role for local diagnosis and assessment for these conditions linked by telecommunications and sharing guidelines and staff with the hospitals.

In many cases, care can be more appropriately given in units providing intermediate care, which need not necessarily be attached to a general hospital. Once again, this makes it possible to provide care in settings that are more accessible for patients and their families. But, as with emergency departments, there are consequences for what is left behind. The patients that do require to be admitted to medical units in hospitals will, on average, be very much sicker, so that much higher staffing levels per patient will be required.

[Third], . . . there is a need to rethink whether emergency medicine and surgery need to be provided together. It may also mean that more surgery will take place in ambulatory centres that are attached to other local services but distant from the main hospital. The separation of planned from unplanned work may also have advantages in terms of reducing the disruption to elective care caused by emergency pressure.

But arguably the surgery, medicine, radiology and other empires that have typified the internal structure of hospitals will soon be obsolete, giving way to an organisation based on body systems, disease groups or shared expertise. Unfortunately, the internal configuration of the hospital – another under-researched area – is slow to follow . . .

The outpatient clinic is the shop window of the hospital. It is also the part that is often least well organised. In many cases management is reactive, with little thought about how processes could be streamlined or coordinated. There is enormous scope for change simply by identifying the common conditions seen in a particular clinic and deciding how they can most efficiently be managed. Major gains are also available by standardising care, 'one-stop' clinics and systematically redesigning the system to make best use of expertise across the whole local health care system, including nurses, therapists, general practitioners and others.

Many of these organisational changes are being driven by the emergence of new technologies. These will have an especially large impact on activities such as imaging and pathology. Whereas previously technology drove centralisation, the likelihood is that near-patient testing kits, mobile radiology facilities and telemedicine will facilitate further dispersion of services.

So what will the hospital of the future look like? Perhaps the only thing of which we can be certain is that it will be different from the hospital of today. The observations above are based on the situation that already exists, but few hospitals being built today take full account of them. As the pace of change quickens, the future is ever more difficult to predict.

Nevertheless, we need to change our vision of what a hospital is and include in our thinking some radically different models of providing health care. Whatever we plan today will be inappropriate for future needs, but we should at least ensure that whatever we do can adapt to changing circumstances with the least amount of difficulty.

 Feedback

1 The authors identify several factors that are leading to a reappraisal of the role of a hospital:

- technological advances such as telemedicine, near-patient testing, day surgery
- patients desire to be treated nearer their homes (i.e. in primary care)
- the development of protocols for the investigation and treatment of common conditions
- avoidance of inappropriate usage such as minor injuries in major emergency departments.

2 They suggest several likely changes:

- fewer hospitals handling major trauma plus local minor injury facilities
- ambulatory surgery centres
- fewer admissions of patients needing assessment and diagnosis
- internal reorganisation of hospitals to make them more patient-centred and less pro-vider (specialty) centred.

The common thread that unites most of these predictions is the shift of health care from hospitals to primary care. In the future it is likely that in all countries you will see fewer hospitals concentrating on the most severely ill patients who require expensive, high technology interventions. Between these and primary care, there will be inter-mediate facilities providing residential or inpatient care for those who have been in the major hospitals but are not yet ready to go home and for those needing inpatient care but are not so ill as to require the services of a major hospital.

Summary

An important aspect of health care reforms in high income countries is the restructuring of health services at institutional level. In this chapter you have looked at management strategies to substitute more appropriate forms for less appropriate forms of care. Substitution is related to changes in type of institution, technology, and staff and skills mix. This goes along with a changing role of hospitals and increased capacities of primary care. Related changes can be observed in the development of human resources in the field of health care.

References

Buchan J, Dal Poz MR (2002). Skill mix in the health care workforce; reviewing the evidence. *Bulletin of the WHO* 80: 575–80.

Edwards N, McKee M (2002). The future role of the hospital. *Journal of Health Services Research & Policy* 7: 1–2.

WHO (2000) *World Health Report*. Geneva: WHO.

SECTION 6

Quality improvement

18 | Defining good quality health services

Overview

This is the first of three chapters on improving the quality of health services. In this chapter you will first learn about the key dimensions of quality and the main steps in quality improvement. The rest of the chapter focuses on the first step, that of defining what practitioners should be doing in terms of policies and clinical practice. You will learn about how the available research evidence should be used and, then, how it can be combined with professional experience using consensus development methods to create guidelines. The following two chapters will consider how the performance of health services can be assessed and how practice and policy can be changed.

Learning objectives

After working through this chapter, you will be better able to:

- describe the dimensions of quality
- outline the quality improvement cycle as a constant process of assessing, monitoring and implementing quality
- describe how the research evidence can be synthesized
- describe how consensus development methods can be used to develop clinical guidelines

Key terms

Audit Review of performance usually judged against agreed criteria and standards.

Clinical guidelines Advice based on the best available research evidence and clinical experience.

Consensus development A set of explicit formal methods for developing and establishing the collective views of a group when faced with uncertainty.

Quality criteria Statements that describe what constitutes good quality care.

Quality improvement A systematic approach to assessing, monitoring and improving performance of health services according to defined standards.

Quality of care The extent to which care is effective, humane and equitable.

Quality standards The desired level of compliance with a quality criterion.

Systematic review A review of the literature that uses an explicit approach to searching, selecting and combining the relevant studies.

What is quality?

'Quality' and 'quality of care' are terms that are used by almost everyone involved in health care. You will find references to quality in many articles and books you read. And you could be forgiven for being unsure what the authors mean, as it is a term that is used rather vaguely.

 Activity 18.1

One simple way of understanding what the word 'quality' means is to define what you mean by a high quality health service. So, complete the sentence: 'A high quality health service would provide care that is . . .'.

 Feedback

A high quality health service would provide care that is effective (the benefits outweigh any possible danger or harm), provided in a humane way (treats people with respect and is timely) and is equitable (available to everyone in need regardless of their sex, age, ethnicity, etc.). Note that this definition does not include any consideration of the other key attribute, cost or efficiency. The challenge for health care policy makers and managers is to provide good quality care at a reasonable cost.

To summarize, the four attributes are:

- *effectiveness* – does the intervention achieve the intended benefit?
- *equity* – is the intervention available to all who could benefit from it?
- *humanity* – is care acceptable to patients?
- *Efficiency* – is care provided in a way that ensures the greatest benefit at least cost?

It is not possible to maximize all four attributes of health services. For example, if you wanted to achieve equity of access to care (e.g. everyone has a health centre within 1 kilometre of their home), the health system would be very expensive (as there would have to be health centres even in remote areas with just a few scattered homesteads). So equity would only be achieved by sacrificing efficiency. Similar trade-offs occur between all four attributes. This is why it cannot be left to experts to decide on the format of a health system but decisions must be taken by politicians who have to consider explicitly the value they put on each attribute. In many ways, the decision a society has to make is not 'what are the features we want in our system' but 'what are the shortcomings that we can accept and put up with (e.g. some lack of equity to ensure greater efficiency).'

Before moving on, there is a fifth attribute that has largely been neglected (particularly in high income countries) – that of sustainability. You could argue that health services cannot be said to be of high quality if they are unstable and difficult to maintain (e.g. unable to recruit and retain appropriate staff). This is not traditionally included in considerations of quality but should not be ignored.

What is quality improvement?

Quality improvement is a systematic approach to achieving agreed standards of care. As shown in Figure 18.1, it is a *continuous process or cycle* involving selecting a topic, establishing criteria of good quality, setting standards, assessing quality and implementing change.

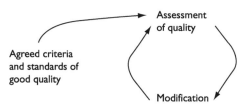

Figure 18.1 Quality improvement cycle

(Source: London School of Hygiene & Tropical Medicine staff)

The first stage is *topic selection*. The more specific and narrowly defined the topic, the more likely you will be able to produce some improvement in quality. For example, it would be better to try and improve the delivery of measles immunization than to take on the challenge of improving the whole of community health services for children.

When selecting a topic, you also need to choose an intervention or activity which is known to be of benefit. You will learn about how to review and synthesize the scientific evidence about the effectiveness and cost-effectiveness of health care later in this chapter.

Having selected your topic, you need to *establish criteria* of good quality. These are statements or objectives of what constitutes good quality. For example, suppose your topic is appendicectomy because you are concerned that the local surgeons are doing unnecessary operations (i.e. operating on people who turn out not to have appendicitis). One criterion might be 'Appendixes that are removed are inflamed'.

Criteria might relate to the structure (input), process or outcome of care. In addition, they need to be objective, measurable and to be acceptable to the health care staff involved in providing the particular service. (You learned about objective measures in Chapter 12.)

Structure measurements are the most basic measure of input, such as the number of staff, professional skills and facilities. Process measures reflect, for example, transport times of car accident victims to hospital, referral rates to tertiary care, waiting times in outpatient departments. And, as you have seen, outcomes are less easy to measure and include such aspects as patient satisfaction with outcome, psychosocial functioning, pain reduction or infection rates.

Activity 18.2

Suggest a structural, process and outcome criterion for appendicectomy.

Feedback

You might have suggested:

structure – operations are carried out by surgeons with 20 years' experience

process – appendixes removed are inflamed

outcome – patients are back to full activity within 4 weeks.

While the ultimate goal of appendicectomy is the outcome, it is generally easier and cheaper to use a process or structural criterion. This is only justified if you know that such criteria are directly associated with good outcomes. In this example you would have to know that surgeons with 20 years' experience achieve better outcomes than less experienced surgeons. If that wasn't the case, then the criterion would not be acceptable.

You may be aware that sometimes patients can appear to have appendicitis but at operation the appendix looks normal. However, if surgeons are very cautious and seek to avoid such 'unnecessary' operations, they will inevitably fail to operate on some patients who do have appendicitis. Such patients' lives will be at risk from untreated appendicitis. So in quality improvement it is necessary to take into account that health care is an inexact science. The way this is done is by *setting standards*, that is, the level of compliance with a criterion. In the example of 'Appendixes removed are inflamed', you might chose to set a standard of 75% compliance (i.e. at least three quarters of appendixes removed will be inflamed). Standards might be set by individual surgeons for themselves, locally by a hospital or nationally (by a surgical organization, a purchaser or a payer). The level at which standards are set will depend on the way the health care system is organized and governed.

Having agreed a standard for each and every criterion, the *quality of the service needs to be assessed*. Ideally, existing sources of information can be used. But if there are none available, special data collection will need to be set up.

If the quality assessment reveals that the service is not achieving the desired level of quality, it is necessary to understand the reasons. There is a natural tendency to respond to a finding of low quality care by providing additional training or refresher education for staff. Sometimes this will be appropriate but it does assume the cause of the problem is that staff don't know what they should be doing. This rarely is the case. The vast majority of instances of poor quality care arise from poor organization of services (and secondly, from inappropriate attitudes towards patients). And the best way, initially, to find out why poor quality exists is to talk to those providing the service. It is essential to consult not only the leading members of staff but also those in supporting roles, such as receptionists and porters. Often the 'discovery' of a quality problem will not be a surprise to those involved and, if you're lucky, the staff will also be able to advise on how it can be corrected.

Having said that, there are plenty of instances where the staff will not know the best way of organizing services and treating patients. One approach, used throughout the world, is to refer to guidelines – expert advice about good quality care. The rest of this chapter is devoted to how guidelines are created. You will learn more about assessing quality in Chapter 19 and more about how to intervene to improve quality in Chapter 20.

Developing guidelines – preparation

Before embarking on creating new guidelines it is vital that you find out if some relevant and applicable guidelines already exist. There are hundreds of guidelines in existence and the number is increasing rapidly throughout the world. For example, the National Guideline Clearinghouse (www.guideline.gov) in the USA had included over 1100 in 2004. Guidelines are produced by a variety of organizations: international agencies; governments; health insurance companies; professional associations; and local groups.

 Activity 18.3

What criteria would you use to decide whether an existing guideline is suitable for your purposes?

 Feedback

The sorts of issues you might have considered are as follows:

1 Is it up-to-date? Research evidence accumulates rapidly in some fields.

2 Is it relevant to my country? Guidelines have to be relevant to the context in which they are going to be adopted, such as the level of health care expenditure or religious beliefs.

3 Is it of good quality? Has it been developed using accepted methods, such as incorporating the available research evidence?

4 Will it be credible or acceptable to local policy-makers and practitioners? Are the developers well respected? Did the developers have any conflict of interest?

Having established that a new guideline needs to be developed, you need to go through several preliminary steps. First, you need to determine who should be involved. There are two groups to consider: the policy-makers or practitioners whose views and behaviour you want the guidelines to influence; and those who will be subject to those views and behaviour (for clinical guidelines that will be patients and their carers; for organizational guidelines it will also include health care staff). The size of the guideline development group will depend on the development method you adopt, and vice versa. Generally, groups are 10–20 in size. Many additional people can be consulted about general or specific issues during the process. Having decided, say, that you want three community health workers to be involved, you have to identify and select specific individuals. They can be randomly or carefully chosen – research suggests that the important factor is a person's 'tribe' (e.g. community health worker) rather than the choice of a particular representative.

Second, having assembled your group, each member needs to declare their beliefs about the topic (e.g. 'the treatment is excellent and should always be used'). They should also declare any potential conflict of interest (e.g. a surgeon who earns money doing a certain procedure which is the subject of the guideline). There is no problem in members having strong beliefs or interests as long as the group, and later on the users of the guideline, are aware of it.

Third, the group need to decide which particular aspects of the guideline topic they are going to focus on. Generally, there are many aspects that could be considered, too many to undertake. So the group must prioritize those areas where they believe guidelines could have the maximum effect on improving the quality of health care, For example, it might be the way patients are investigated and diagnosed rather than how best to treat them or how best to help them rehabilitate afterwards.

The process of defining precisely the scope of the guidelines will need to take into account whether or not any good quality research evidence exists. So the process has to be iterative. After a preliminary prioritization, it will be necessary to see what research evidence exists. The final decision on scope will be arrived at by considering the group's priorities in the light of the availability of research evidence.

Reviewing the research evidence

The first thing to do is to check whether anyone else has already reviewed the literature. To be acceptable, a review needs to have adopted clear methods for:

- searching the literature
- selecting potential papers
- judging the methodological quality of the studies
- synthesizing the evidence from all the papers selected.

The outcome of such a process is known as a *systematic review*. While it was developed primarily to consider quantitative research evidence on the effectiveness of health care interventions, it has been developed to encompass economic evaluations and evidence from qualitative studies. (It is not so appropriate for reviewing theoretical or methodological topics.)

As with guidelines, there is a rapidly growing number of systematic reviews available. One source is the Database of Abstracts of Reviews of Effects (DARE) which includes structured abstracts of systematic reviews from around the world, which have been critically appraised by reviewers (www.york.ac.uk/inst/crd/darehp.htm). For inclusion, reviews must meet at least three of the following four criteria, of which criteria 1 and 2 are mandatory:

1 Were inclusion/exclusion criteria reported that addressed the review question? A good review should focus on a well defined question, which defines the inclusion/exclusion criteria by which decisions are made on whether to include or exclude primary studies. The criteria should relate to the four components of study design, participants, intervention or organization, and outcomes of interest.

2 Was the search adequate? This is usually the case if details of electronic database searches and other identification strategies are given. Ideally, details of the search terms used, date and language restrictions should be presented. In addition, descriptions of hand-searching, attempts to identify unpublished material, and any contact with authors, industry, and research institutes should be provided. The appropriateness of the database(s) searched by the authors

should also be considered – for example, if MEDLINE is searched for a review evaluating health promotion, then it is unlikely that all relevant studies will have been located.

3 Was the validity of the included studies assessed? Authors should have taken account of study design and quality, either by restricting inclusion criteria, or systematic assessment of study quality. A systematic assessment of the quality of primary studies should include information about the criteria used (e.g. method of randomization, whether outcome assessment was blinded). Authors often use a published checklist or scale, or one that they have designed specifically for their review.

4 Are sufficient details about the individual included studies presented? The review should demonstrate that the studies included are suitable to answer the question posed and that a judgement on the appropriateness of the authors' conclusions can be made.

These criteria also serve as advice as to how you should go about your own systematic review if no existing ones are suitable. For more detail as to how to conduct a review, you should consult one of the many instruction manuals available. You will find a free one at www.york.ac.uk/inst/crd/crd4_content.pdf.

Developing guidelines – combining research evidence with experience

Occasionally in health care there is clear research evidence to indicate the best way of managing a patient or organizing a service. Generally, however, the research evidence is either lacking or of poor quality. Even when the research evidence is of reasonable quality, there is a need to translate it into guidelines for a particular place. That is because the local context must be considered. The latter includes the level of resources, the skill of staff, and the beliefs and attitudes of the local population. You have already seen in Chapter 8 the impact such factors can have. Savoie *et al.* (2000) compared five guidelines for cholesterol testing. Three had been developed in Canada, one in the USA and one in the UK. All five development groups reviewed the same literature and drew the same conclusions from it. However, the five sets of recommendations differed significantly in several respects, including who should be screened:

- UK: no one should be screened
- Canada (A): men aged 30–59 years
- Canada (B): men aged 45–75 years
- Canada (C): men aged 40–70 years and women aged 50–70 years
- USA: men and women aged over 20 years.

Given the differences between the three Canadian guidelines, there must be factors other than the local context causing the variation in guidance. The authors felt the key factor was the way the opinions and experience of clinicians were combined with the research evidence in the group. Traditionally this has been done by a group of self-appointed 'experts' forming a committee and making decisions in an informal way (without any explicit rules).

Activity 18.4

Think about any committees you have been on. What do you think are the dangers of an informal process for decision-making?

 Feedback

There are several dangers in relying on an informal process: the most powerful members of the group often dominate and the less confident or less powerful feel unable to challenge; the reasons for decisions may not be clear; the group is more likely to arrive at inconsistent decisions.

These concerns have led to the use of formal *consensus development methods*. Of the several methods available, the most commonly used one for developing guidelines is the nominal group technique (Black *et al.* 1999). It has several forms but the key common features are that the group members express their views in private so they should not feel under any pressure from other members and that the group meet at least once to discuss the more controversial issues and to learn the reasons for any areas of disagreement. While the aim is to improve the level of agreement within the group, there should be no attempt to pressurise members to agree just for the sake of it.

Summary

You have seen that quality has three key dimensions – effectiveness, equity and humanity – and the aim of all health care systems is to maximize the quality of care given the resources available. You have learned about the stages of the quality improvement cycle and then focused on the first two stages, selecting a topic and establishing criteria of good quality care. In the next chapter you will go on to learn about setting standards and assessing performance.

References

Black NA, Murphy M, Lamping D, McKee M, Sanderson C, Askham J *et al.* (1999). Consensus development methods: a review of best practice in creating clinical guidelines. *Journal of Health Services Research & Policy* 4: 236–44.

Savoie I, Kazanjian A, Bassett K (2000). Do clinical practice guidelines reflect research evidence? *Journal of Health Services Research & Policy* 5: 76–82.

19 Performance assessment

Overview

In the previous chapter you learned about the dimensions of quality and the stages of the quality improvement cycle. You went on to learn about how criteria of good quality can be derived from reviewing the research literature and combining that with the views of relevant stakeholders such as clinicians and lay people. In this chapter you will learn about the next stages, setting standards and assessing performance. In Chapter 20 you will complete the quality improvement journey by considering what action can be taken to improve quality.

Learning objectives

After working through this chapter, you will be better able to:

- **understand the importance to health services of maintaining public trust**
- **describe the relative advantages of measuring inputs, processes or outcomes**
- **understand the steps involved in making meaningful comparisons of providers**
- **discuss how performance data should be disclosed to the public.**

Key terms

Case mix The mix of cases (or patients) that a provider cares for.

Iatrogenesis Disease resulting from medical or health care interventions.

Risk (case-mix) adjustment A statistical process to make allowance for any difference in case mix between providers when comparing their performance.

Trust and accountability

Before considering how the performance of health services can be assessed, it is important to pause and consider why it is felt necessary to invest so many resources in scrutinizing performance. In essence, it is necessary because the public cannot assume that all is well just because health care professionals say so. In other words, the public and patients cannot automatically trust professionals.

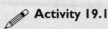 **Activity 19.1**

There is evidence that the level of public trust has fallen over recent years in high income countries, a view expressed by Huw Davies (1999) in the following article. As you read it, consider the following questions:

1 What does the author mean by 'public trust'?
2 How can accountability be achieved?

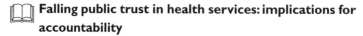 **Falling public trust in health services: implications for accountability**

The barrage of adverse reports about health care cannot but affect public confidence in health care professionals and the quality of the services they deliver. Indeed, one of the major themes to emerge from contemplation of the Bristol case [in which two surgeons continued to operate despite mounting concerns], by both professional and lay commentators, was the damage that such cases do to public trust and the need for more effective accountability of health care professionals. In the USA too there is deepening concern about falling public trust in a wide range of public institutions, health care organisations among them. The private sector fares no better in the public eye and managed care in particular provokes strong feelings of concern and mistrust.

Yet what is public trust? In the literature, definitions differ but all embody the notion of expectations: expectations by the public that health care providers will demonstrate knowledge, skill and competence; further expectations too that they will behave as true agents (that is, in the patient's best interest) and with beneficence, fairness and integrity. It is these collective expectations that form the basis of trust, and these same expectations that can be shaken by repeated demonstrations that all is not well with health care. Trust is slowly gained but easily lost in the face of confounded expectations.

We should not underestimate the potential importance of falling public trust in health services. Although unfounded trust is merely hope and dependency (and its loss may be no loss at all), a robust public trust may be advantageous in many ways. Social commentators such as Francis Fukuyama have attempted to explain differential national economic performance and prosperity by reference to natural variations in trust. Thus trust is seen as a kind of 'social capital' which allows efficient smooth-running relationships with small overheads. Without trust we may have to turn to new ways of defining relationships. These new ways of managing relationships may in turn have further impact on trust. One of the key relationships on which public trust may have impact is the 'accountability relationship' between the public and various health care organisations.

The public have a right to expect that health care organisations will operate effectively. To some extent, and this varies between countries, such expectations are taken on trust. However, when trust is damaged, the public seeks new routes to accountability . . .

Accountability can be achieved by a number of different routes. First, organisations can provide formal accounts (such as annual reports) of their mission, objectives, activities and progress. Such accounts may, however, be seen as mainly 'public relations', putting a good gloss on things and serving a largely ceremonial role. Thus, in health care, these general accounts are increasingly supplemented by the publication of specific performance data on a wide range of dimensions. In the USA, HEDIS Data (Health Plan Employer Data and Information Set) report on the performance of health plans (purchasers), and a plethora of 'report cards' furnish information on providers. In the UK, the National Performance Framework seeks to develop explicit reporting of performance and national comparisons on a wide scale . . .

. . . Each approach to accountability has its own area of application, and its own advantages, costs and burdens. With all the approaches there is scope for perverse incentives and dysfunctional consequences (undesirable changes in behaviour in response to the account-ability system). In addition, there is some concern that changing emphases on external accountability might exert influence on mechanisms of governance within organisations in less than desirable ways. Most developed nations use an ever-shifting mix of these different systems, as an over-reliance on any single approach tends merely to highlight its flaws. Further, the routine application of many of the approaches to accountability may lead to ritualistic rather than instrumental systems.

. . . Before trust as a basis for the relationship between the public and their health care services is further undermined, we should begin to identify how public trust sustains well-functioning organisations – especially those agencies in the public sector that lack market discipline.

We also need a much clearer idea of whether and how too much trust shields the incompetent. Finally, we still have only the vaguest ideas about what nurtures public trust in the first place or impacts adversely upon it. The role of the media may be crucial here, but this and other factors – such as the rise of the consumer and the decline of the professional – need to be examined both theoretically and empirically.

 Feedback

1 'Public trust' embodies the notion of the expectations the public have that clinicians will be knowledgeable, skilful, competent; that they will behave in the patient's best interest with beneficence, fairness and integrity.

2 Accountability can be achieved through formal accounts (e.g. annual reports) and the publication of performance data, backed up by methods of regulation such as accreditation. (You will learn more about such methods in Chapter 20.)

Methods of assessing performance

Performance assessment is not new. The use of quantitative measures was under-taken by Florence Nightingale when she compared London hospitals in the nineteenth century and was continued by two surgeons in the early twentieth century – EW Groves in Bristol, England, and EA Codman in Boston, USA. You saw in Chapter 2 how, by the 1980s, Arnold Relman considered that a new era of assessment and accountability had arrived centre stage.

Activity 19.2

Remind yourself of the reasons Relman gave for the current focus on assessment and accountability.

Feedback

He cited several factors, including:

- the need for cost containment
- advances in health care technology producing new opportunities and ways of delivering care
- evidence of wide variations in the use of health care between geographical populations.

Since then, there has also been a growing awareness of the incidence of iatrogenesis (harm caused by health care). In addition, the rapid development of the Internet has meant that members of the public have gained access to lots of medical information resulting in much better informed, and in some cases more critical, patients and their carers.

The last few years have seen a huge growth in the use of quantitative measures of performance. Assessment may be at the micro level of individual clinicians or groups of clinicians in departments or units, at the meso level of organizations (health centres, hospitals), or at the macro level of entire health care systems.

Assessment may involve scrutiny of the inputs (structures) to health care, the processes of care, or the outcomes of care. Choice of the type of measure involves a trade-off. Ultimately, what the public are concerned about is outcomes – whether you are more or less likely to survive or get better with one provider rather than another. However, as you have seen in Chapter 12, measurement and collection of data on outcomes can be complex and expensive. At the other extreme, measures of inputs are cheap and easy to acquire but may not provide a valid indication of performance. For example, the mere fact that a nurse has certain qualifications doesn't automatically mean he or she is a good performer whose patients do well.

In the middle are process measures which are easier to collect than outcomes and do not involve any delay in waiting to see the patient's outcome. While they are often the best option, process measures are only valid if they correlate closely with outcomes. For example, it is well recognized that people who have suffered a heart attack are more likely to survive if they are treated with thrombolytic (clot-busting) drugs. It is, therefore, legitimate to assess the performance of health services for people with heart disease by measuring the proportion of heart attack victims who receive these drugs promptly. In contrast, many countries use the rate of patient readmissions to hospital as a measure of quality of care. The problem is that a readmission rate appears to have no or little association with valid outcome measures. (This should not be a surprise given that admission rates vary considerably due to variations in clinical judgement – see Chapter 8.)

The key elements of any performance assessment, regardless of the level of analysis (micro, meso, macro) or the use of process or outcome measures are:

- definition of the variable being measured
- data collection
- case-mix or risk adjustment for meaningful comparisons
- presentation and dissemination of comparisons.

Each step presents potential difficulties for the unwary. You have already seen in Chapter 17 that even apparently straightforward variables may prove difficult to define.

 Activity 19.3

What difficulties do you think you might encounter in defining the following?

1 A breast-fed infant
2 Diabetes
3 Length of hospital stay
4 High quality food for inpatients.

 Feedback

1 You would need to define whether you meant exclusively breast-fed or not. Would once a day for a few minutes count as 'breast-fed'?

2 While some conditions are either present or not (e.g. a broken bone), most occur in a wide spectrum of severity from mild and insignificant to severe and life-threatening. To lump together such diverse cases may be misleading.

3 Length of stay can be defined as starting on arrival at a hospital or arrival on a ward; some hospitals will count a day-case staying 8 hours as 'one day', whereas others may not include them as 'admissions'.

4 Need to develop criteria such as nutritional content, temperature of hot food, taste, etc.

The problems of collecting data may be more familiar to you. It is almost inevitable that some data will be missing. If this occurs randomly and only occasionally, then it is unlikely to matter. But in some health care systems, missing data are so common as to render the data unfit for assessing performance. The other problem is the validity of the data. There is some evidence that data may be deliberately distorted by providers to ensure their performance appears good. Such 'gaming', if widespread, could undermine the validity of the assessments.

As you will be aware, the types of patients different doctors and different institutions care for vary. Sometimes this is deliberate. For example, tertiary care facilities are expected to manage particularly complex and difficult cases. If doctors' or institutions' performance were to be compared without taking such differences into account, the comparisons would at best be meaningless and at worst misleading. The performance measure (be it process or outcome) needs to take the *different mix of cases* each provider manages (case mix) into account by statistical adjustment. This is also referred to as 'risk adjustment' (as you are adjusting for each patient's risk of a good or bad outcome).

Activity 19.4

Adjusting for all relevant characteristics of patients is challenging. Why do you think that is so?

 Feedback

You need to take into account and adjust for every patient characteristic that might be associated with the performance measure (e.g. survival, length of stay). That presupposes that all the relevant characteristics are known and can be measured. While some are well recognized, such as age (generally the older a patient, the worse their outcome), others may be unknown. Sometimes a characteristic might be suspected, such as personality, but not easily measured on a routine basis.

Concern about the difficulties of case-mix adjustment, together with fears about 'gaming the system', has led some commentators to reject the use of performance measures. Their concerns extend to claims that such assessments will also cause providers to change their practices in ways that may disadvantage some patients. The commonest example cited is that providers stop treating very sick patients who have a poor prognosis as the death of such patients will harm the providers' assessment. This and other concerns are addressed in the following edited article by Edward Hannan (1998) who pioneered the development and introduction of performance assessment of cardiac surgeons in New York State in the early 1990s.

 Activity 19.5

As you read the following, make notes on what the three criticisms of the New York State approach have been and what Hannan's response is.

 Measuring hospital outcomes: don't make perfect the enemy of good!

In recent years there has been a proliferation of outcomes research in an attempt to measure the quality of health care. One of the types that has been most popular, and most controversial, is the development and sometimes public dissemination of risk-adjusted adverse outcome rates (usually mortality) for surgical procedures or medical conditions.

. . . The first public report based on clinical data collected expressly for the purpose of assessing quality was the New York State Cardiac Surgery Report in 1990 (Hannan *et al.* 1990), which was followed by a similar report on cardiac surgery in Pennsylvania that was released in 1992. These reports, which continue to be produced, present risk-adjusted mortality for surgeons who perform coronary artery bypass grafting (CABG) and for hospitals in which CABG is performed . . .

These efforts have been vociferously criticized. Among the reasons given are that the statistical models do not adjust adequately for differences in the pre-operative risks of patients, that the publication of death rates results in perverse incentives regarding treatment decisions that could have adverse consequences for patients, and that public dissemination results subsequently in over-reporting of risk factors by hospitals that yields an inaccurate risk-adjustment process.

Inadequacy of risk adjustment

Some of the justification for maintaining that the models are not good enough is that there are large changes in provider risk-adjusted mortality ranks from year to year. Although this is true, the idea that ranks are an important indication of relative quality is merely an ignorant misconception as to how the information is to be used. Hospitals are judged to have different adverse outcome rates only when their risk-adjusted mortalities are found to be statistically different. In fact most, if not all, of the reports I have seen present the outcomes in alphabetical order of provider, rather than in the order of risk-adjusted mortality, so as to discourage improper use of the data in the reports.

Creation of perverse incentives for providers

The only study I am aware of that addresses perverse incentives regarding treatment decisions is a study that concludes that significantly more high-risk New York State patients migrated out of the state to undergo CABG at the Cleveland Clinic during 1989–1993 than during 1980–1988 (Omoigui et al. 1996). However, the time period being used is inaccurate since New York data were released for the first time in December 1990. Also, the average severity of New York State patients at the Cleveland Clinic changed little between 1990 and 1993. Furthermore, the annual number of patients undergoing CABG in New York rose at a fairly steady pace, as did the average pre-operative severity of these patients. A study using Medicare data (which is the only US national database) demonstrated that the proportion of New York patients referred out-of-state for CABG actually declined from 14.8% in 1989 to 11.8% in 1992.

Over-reporting of risk factors

There are undoubtedly perverse incentives associated with reporting the risk factors used to adjust for case mix in a clinical database that is to be used for public dissemination of information, since the sicker a provider's patients appear, the lower the provider's risk-adjusted mortality will be. However, these incentives can be controlled by monitoring data quality. Contrary to allegations that the reported prevalence rates of risk factors in New York have fluctuated wildly, they have actually remained quite stable except for changes related to new definitions for risk factors (Chassin et al. 1996) . . .

Can risk-adjusted outcomes indicate quality of care?

Concerning the use of risk-adjusted outcomes for improving the quality of health care, Brook et al. (1996) state that, with exceptions, the assessment of quality should rely more on process data than outcome data. The main reason given for this opinion is that outcome data may not be sensitive enough since there is not always a poor outcome whenever there is an error in the provision of care. However, these authors also state that there are exceptions to the rule, such as methods of comparing outcomes following CABG. Among the reasons they give for why this is an exception are that there has been extensive research on the best way to adjust statistically for case-mix differences, there is strong evidence of the link between quality of care and survival, death is a common enough event to be used as a measure of quality differences, and differences in mortality between providers (hospitals and surgeons) can be assessed relatively soon after surgery.

I agree with this assessment and commend Brook *et al.* for delineating these factors. Furthermore, I believe that there are many acute medical conditions (such as acute myocardial infarction, stroke, pneumonia, congestive heart failure) and surgical procedures (such as angioplasty, carotid endarterectomy, bowel surgery, hip replacement, back surgery) that meet the conditions mentioned by Brook *et al.*, particularly if death and/or major complications is used as an adverse outcome measure instead of just death.

Also, it is not always known what the optimal processes of care are that lead to better outcomes. The only way to establish this is by observing care with and without what are thought to be optimal processes and demonstrating that the processes lead to better (risk-adjusted) outcomes. After this has been done, it may or may not be advisable to abandon the effort of generating risk-adjusted outcomes.

Conclusions

It is essential that the health services research community continues to improve on hospital and physician quality assessments. There are many areas we need to address, including the theory underlying the statistical models, data quality and accuracy, and preventing or minimizing perverse incentives caused by public release . . . However, there is simply not enough evidence to discontinue these reports, particularly the ones based on clinical data. The best and fastest way to improve them is to search for constructive changes and alternatives while continuing the reports.

 Feedback

The three criticisms and Hannan's responses are as follows:

1 Large fluctuations in ranking of hospitals is evidence of inadequate risk adjustment. In response, Hannan points out that ranking is indeed a very unstable indicator and one that shouldn't be used.

2 The approach creates perverse incentives for providers such as driving high risk patients out of the system. Hannan shows that the severity of cases treated outside New York State did not change and the proportion who migrated out actually fell.

3 Gaming the system by over-reporting patient severity. Hannan states that there is little evidence of this happening; it should be monitored and, if detected, severe sanctions taken.

Performance assessment in low and middle income countries

Most of the discussion of performance assessment so far has implicitly been oriented to high income countries with widespread availability of computer-based data collection. But it would be wrong to conclude that the performance of health services in low and middle income countries is not possible. The following is an extract from an article by Lynne Franco *et al.* (2002) based on their experience of assessing quality in Malawi. They comment on the strengths and weaknesses of four common assessment methods.

Methods for assessing quality of provider performance in developing countries

Observation of provider performance using a checklist

Observation is generally considered as a gold standard for other assessment methods, although there appear to be few empirical studies to validate this. Information derived from observation, when recorded on a structured checklist simultaneously with the provider's actions by an independent observer, provides one of the most complete and reliable pictures of what providers do. This method does not rely on the provider's or the client's memory. However, observers may be unable to discern performance of mental tasks, such as using information collected during history and physical examination of the patient to reach a diagnosis. In addition, observed performance may not represent routine performance if providers modify their behavior while being observed, and providers may not perform in a consistent manner with every patient they encounter.

Exit interviews with patients or caretakers about provider performance

The reliability of exit interview data depends on the memory of the patient or caretaker, how much attention was paid to the provider's actions, knowledge, and expectations about what the provider should be doing, and comfort with talking to an interviewer. However, if conducted without provider knowledge, exit interviews may capture routine performance. Such interviews could provide a clinically trained interviewer with the opportunity to re-examine the patient to assess accuracy of the diagnosis, although such an examination would add time and other costs to this method, and have some of its own methodological problems.

Reviewing patient or health facility records to assess provider performance

Record reviews, commonly used in industrialized countries, allow retrospective assessment of routine provider performance. Limited only by availability and quality of data, record review can assess a large number of cases, and enables review of severely ill cases or rarer conditions. Yet. in developing countries, medical records rarely record findings used to make a diagnosis or any instructions given to the patient. In many outpatient settings, if any records are maintained, they either go home with the patient (e.g. immunization cards or Under-Five cards, etc.) or are health center patient registers that record only the patient's age, sex, domicile, diagnosis, and treatment given.

Interviews with providers about their performance

Provider interviews or self-reports supply information about what providers know, not necessarily what they routinely do. They can, however, furnish information about how providers interpret information from the history and physical examination of the patient. and how they would manage severe cases or referrals.

The formulation of interview questions will also affect the results obtained. Spontaneous responses to open-ended questions (e.g. 'What questions do you ask a patient presenting with cough?') are likely to underestimate what providers do, both for tasks they do not perform often, and for tasks they perform so often that performance becomes unconscious. Probing to stimulate memory or providing fixed choices on self-report can also stimulate responses corresponding to what the provider thinks is the expected answer.

Public reporting of performance

Hannan stresses the need for even greater data accuracy if the results are going to be made public. And if trust in health services is to be maintained and even increased, public dissemination must inevitably occur. Few countries have gone as far as the USA yet so it is to that country that we must turn to see what lessons might be learned from their experience.

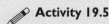 **Activity 19.5**

As you read the following edited article by Martin Marshall *et al.* (2000), consider what the main dangers of public disclosure are perceived to be.

📖 Public reporting of performance: lessons from the USA

Information about the performance of health care providers and health plans has been published in the USA for over a decade . . . This experience provides a useful insight for other countries, where the expansion of public disclosure from its current low levels is advocated by governments as a mechanism to improve accountability and drive quality improvement. Despite the significant differences in culture and health care organisation, much could be gained by studying examples of successful reporting systems and learning from the mistakes that have been made in the USA.

. . . Most fundamentally, the intended purpose or purposes of public disclosure should be made clear to all stakeholders. This is particularly important for health professionals and provider organisations who are likely to question the resources that they will have to expend on the collection and reporting of performance information. The intended purpose will dictate the content and process of release as well as the evaluation criteria used to assess whether and how public disclosure is improving quality of care. In the USA, the primary rationale articulated for public disclosure has been the empowerment of informed consumers, but there is little evidence that this has been realised to any significant extent (Schneider and Epstein 1998). Other important reasons, such as promoting health care improvements, have not been as clearly articulated until recently. It is hoped that the publication of performance information will encourage (or, where appropriate, shame) providers to focus on quality improvement through internal mechanisms rather than through external market forces. Public dissemination of the information is partly a response to the disappointing level of improvement resulting from the use of internal audit data (Davis *et al.* 1995). Certainly, the evidence from the USA suggests that provider organisations, rather than consumers or individual health professionals, are the key audience for information about performance. This reflects the sensitivity of these organisations to their public image, their authority and their ability to implement directly actions that may remedy levels of performance.

Public disclosure should be seen as an evolutionary process becoming progressively more sophisticated and comprehensive over time. Data for public release do not have to be perfect but do have to be good enough to achieve a 'buy-in' from the various stakeholders. For example, the High Level Performance Indicators in England may be regarded as an acceptable starting point, but their selection, measurement and reporting will need to be refined year-on-year if credibility is to be achieved and maintained . . .

Health professionals and their representative bodies should play a significant part in the process of public disclosure. Successful examples of public disclosure in the USA, such as the New York Cardiac Surgery Reporting System, have worked closely with clinicians from the start. Some reporting systems have allowed professionals and organisations a period of time to respond to the performance data and to put mechanisms into place to improve performance prior to publication. Others have encouraged written responses to the data, which are published alongside the performance reports. In return, clinicians should begin to regard public disclosure as a professional responsibility and a core component of the accountability for continuous quality improvement.

Specific educational initiatives should be implemented alongside the performance reports. This would increase the chances of a constructive response and reduce the risk of the misinformed or defensive response that has been observed to several reporting systems in the USA. Educational packages should be targeted at each of the stakeholders. In particular, education of the media has proven to be an important component of successful reporting in the USA. In addition, accompanying comparative performance reports with expert analysis and interpretation could help providers to make the most effective use of the data.

Public disclosure should be accompanied by a strategy for monitoring not only the benefits but also the risks and unintended consequences. Publication of deficiencies in the care provided by professionals who already feel overburdened can be demoralising and may adversely effect public trust in the health service. This is particularly important in publicly funded health systems, where there may be fewer opportunities to exercise choice than in the USA. Misinterpretation of information, manipulation of data and an inappropriate focus on what is being measured, to the detriment of other areas of activity, have all been described (Smith 1995). Some of these effects are inevitable, but the US experience suggests that they can be predicted and managed to optimise the benefits of public disclosure. Alongside the potential benefits, the financial costs of implementing a national policy need to be considered. There has been no accurate assessment of the costs in the USA, but the resources required to develop indicators, measure, report and most importantly act on sub-optimal performance are likely to be significant. The opportunity costs of allocating resources to these processes, in place of direct patient care, need to be defended.

. . . Both the benefits and the problems of transferring ideas between different health systems have been well described. The US experience of public disclosure is a prime example of a health policy initiative that has lessons for other countries. They would do well to heed these lessons and not attempt to re-invent the wheel.

 Feedback

Three potential dangers are identified: the risk of demoralizing providers by 'naming and shaming' them; damage to public trust; and wasting resources on an activity of unproven benefit.

Single indices of performance

At the end of the twentieth century, some countries and international bodies adopted the ambitious objective of trying to develop single over-arching indices that would inform the public about the performance of a provider or a whole system. The idea that the complexity and variability of health care could be reduced to a single rating was one that many observers find naive. Despite this, all health care providers in England were rated on a four point scale (so-called star ratings), and the WHO rated 191 countries' health care systems and then ranked them from 'best' to 'worst'.

There are many problems with such initiatives, not least the inadequacy of the available routine data which, as you have seen in earlier chapters, is rarely fit for this purpose. An even greater problem is how such disparate factors as the cleanliness of a hospital, the waiting time in the emergency room and post-operative mortality can sensibly be bolted together to create a composite index.

The *World Health Report 2000* (WHO 2000) did something similar but at the health system level. The components of its assessment were:

- population health (disability-adjusted life expectancy; child survival)
- responsiveness (respect for people; prompt attention; choice of provider; access to social support networks during care)
- fairness in financial contribution (fraction of disposable income that each household contributes)
- health system efficiency (outcomes achieved per unit of resource used).

Apart from the inadequacy of the available data for many of these indicators, it is not clear why some are even included (e.g. choice of provider). This reveals the ideological values that the developers hold. In addition, the health of a population is only partly a reflection of the performance of its health services – it is more to do with socioeconomic, nutritional and environmental factors. Finally, a country's ranking in the world league table will depend crucially on the relative importance ascribed to the very wide range of indicators included. For example, if population health was considered the most important outcome, you would arrive at a different rank order than if you considered responsiveness as more important.

Does any of this matter? It does if the public release of such rankings leads to unjustified political instability in countries getting a low ranking. What is really needed are performance measures that are accurate, comparisons that are meaningful, and interpretations that enable providers to use the information to improve their services. In other words, performance assessment is not simply a technical challenge but a political, organizational and managerial one. That's what makes it so demanding but also so exciting.

Summary

You have seen how crucial it is that health service providers (and to a lesser extent purchasers) maintain public trust in their services. One approach is to assess their performance using inputs, processes or outcomes. To make meaningful comparisons of performance between providers it is essential to adjust for case-mix differences. Finally, experience is accumulating about how best to disclose performance information to the public.

References

Brook RH, McGlynn EA, Cleary PD (1996). Measuring quality of care. *New England Journal of Medicine* 335: 966–70.

Chassin MR, Hannan EL, DeBuono BA (1996). Benefits and hazards of reporting risk-adjusted outcomes publicly. *New England Journal of Medicine* 334: 394–8.

Davies H (1999). Falling public trust in health services: implications for accountability. *Journal of Health Services Research & Policy* 4: 193–4.

Davis DA, Thomson MA, Oxman AD, Haynes B (1995). Changing physician performance: a systematic review of the effect of continuing medical education strategies. *Journal of the American Medical Association* 274: 700–5.

Franco LM, Franco C, Kumwenda N, Nkhoma W (2002). Methods for assessing quality of provider performance in developing countries. *International Journal of Quality in Health Care* 14(Suppl. 1): 17–24.

Hannan EL (1998). Measuring hospital outcomes: don't make perfect the enemy of good! *Journal of Health Services Research & Policy* 3: 67–9.

Hannan EL, Kilburn H Jr, O'Donnell JF, Lukacik G, Shields EP (1990). Adult open heart surgery in New York State: an analysis of risk factors and hospital mortality rates. *Journal of the American Medical Association* 264: 2768–74.

Marshall M, Shekelle P, Brook R, Leatherman S (2000). Public reporting of performance: lessons from the USA. *Journal of Health Services Research & Policy* 5: 1–2.

Omoigui NA, Miller DP, Brown KJ *et al.* (1996). Outmigration for coronary bypass surgery in an era of public dissemination of clinical outcomes. *Circulation* 93: 27–33.

Schneider EC, Epstein AM (1998). Use of public performance reports: a survey of patients undergoing cardiac surgery. *Journal of the American Medical Association* 279: 1638–42.

Smith P (1995). On the unintended consequences of publishing performance data in the public sector. *International Journal of Public Administration* 18: 277–310.

WHO (2000). *World Health Report*. Geneva: WHO.

20 Improving quality of care

Overview

In the previous two chapters you learned about the dimensions of quality, the stages in the quality improvement cycle, how to establish criteria of good quality care (guidelines), and how to assess quality (or performance) using quantitative measures. You also learned about one particular method of intervening to improve quality, namely the public disclosure of comparative performance. In this final chapter you will learn about the wide variety of interventions available.

Learning objectives

After working through this chapter, you will be better able to:

- **map the available interventions to change services**
- **describe the range of interventions that have been used.**

Key terms

Accreditation A voluntary survey of quality standards, performed by an independent body awarding grades.

Litigation Legal action taken by patients against health care providers for alleged malpractice.

Total quality management (continuous quality improvement) An approach to quality improvement that involves the commitment of all members of an organization to meeting the needs of its external and internal customers.

Mapping quality improvement interventions

A wide variety of interventions are available to improve the quality of health services. Not surprisingly, this panoply of methods often causes confusion for practitioners, managers and policy makers.

 Activity 20.1

Spend a few minutes writing down all the interventions or approaches to ensuring and improving quality that you are aware of in your own country.

Feedback

You may have included some of the following which are commonly used around the world: registration of professionals; accreditation of facilities; clinical audit; accreditation of training facilities; litigation for malpractice; financial incentives; inspectorates; inquiries.

In many countries, quality improvement methods have been introduced gradually, each new one being added to existing activities. The result has been a jungle of uncoordinated activities that can cause confusion, consume excessive resources and antagonize the very people (providers) whose performance you want to improve. As a first step to understanding the contribution of each approach, it is helpful to map the existing terrain (Black 1990). To do this it is necessary to adopt some criteria by which each approach can be assessed. Two particular criteria that have been used are:

1 *Internal versus external*. This considers *where* the approach is conducted. The possibilities extend from self-assessment or audit by individual clinicians (looking critically at their own performance in private, without anyone else involved) to national (or even international) approaches by external organizations such as governments or health insurance companies.

2 *Reactive versus proactive*. This considers *when* the approach is used. There are two possibilities. It may be reactive, that is, it occurs after poor quality has occurred or is suspected, such as an inquiry into why a particular patient had a poor outcome. Alternatively, it may be proactive, routinely assessing quality to detect any sub-optimal care.

✐ **Activity 20.2**

Think about your own country again and try and map onto the grid below the quality improvement approaches of which you are aware.

	External		Internal
	National	District/Unit	Individual
Reactive			
Regular			

Feedback

Table 20.1, which is based on the situation in the UK, illustrates some of the frequently used approaches in health systems around the world.

Table 20.1 Approaches frequently used in health systems

	External		Internal
	National	District/Unit	Individual
Reactive	Medical litigation General Medical Council (Disciplinary)	Clinical meetings	
	Confidential inquiries		
	Performance Indicators		
	Quality control of laboratories		
	Accreditation of training (Royal Colleges)		
	General Medical Council (re-validation)	Accreditation of training (PG dean)	
	National Audit Office		
Regular	Healthcare Commission	Peer review	Self-audit

Before you learn about all the specific interventions available, there is one other aspect to consider – the way in which health care providers use the approaches. Traditionally providers would select a method and carry out a one-off activity. For example, they might decide to review the quality of the food being provided for inpatients or the rate of obstetric mishaps. This would be followed up with an intervention, such as a retraining session or the issuance of guidelines. Since the 1980s, the traditional approach has been challenged by a more ongoing approach in which the whole culture of a provider organization is committed to quality improvement. This is known as *total quality management* (or continuous quality improvement).

This is based on the conviction that high quality services are those that best meet the needs of most customers. While the obvious 'customers' are the patients being served, also included are the internal customers. The latter are staff who depend on the services of other staff (e.g. ward nurses depend on porters to move patients; doctors depend on staff in diagnostic departments to carry out tests). In this approach, quality is the responsibility of all staff, not just those employed to undertake quality improvement. It presupposes that there are clear and proper long term organizational goals which all staff are aware of and committed to. The organization needs to establish good communication throughout so that staff are kept informed of their own performance and achievements. Needless to say, the emphasis is on learning from experiences, supporting those who need assistance and avoiding a blame culture in which staff feel the need to hide any faults through fear of punishment.

So what interventions to improve quality are available? Although, as you have seen, there are many, they can be considered in six categories, each of which you will consider in the rest of this chapter:

- education
- feedback of information
- incentives
- administrative structures and processes
- regulation
- legislation.

Education

Education (or re-education) tends to be the first response following the identification of poor quality care. However, generally staff know what they should be doing. Problems arise when they act differently, for example taking 'short cuts' to speed up their work. Having said that, it may well be appropriate to establish (or re-establish) what everyone should be doing. While there are many ways of educating people, the most frequently used in quality improvement are: meetings or seminars; issuance of guidelines; and, in countries with computing facilities, computer-generated reminders.

You have learned about the development of guidelines in Chapter 18. Guidelines are often fairly extensive documents so it is necessary to create short versions that people will have time to use. It is now standard practice to issue guidelines in three forms: an extensive account providing background information and the evidence on which they are based; a shorter version for the relevant health care workers; and a very short version for patients that avoids jargon and non-essential technical detail.

In high and middle income countries with widespread computing facilities in their health systems, it is possible to build in automatic reminders so that good quality care does not depend on a health care worker having to remember key events. For example, many child health services have a database of all the children they are responsible for such that when a child is due for an immunization or developmental check, the computer lets everyone know. This can help ensure high coverage and reduce the risk of delayed detection of treatable problems.

Feedback of information

Many health care workers are unaware of their own and their organization's performance because they receive no routine information. While simply providing such information may not in itself be sufficient to change behaviour and practice, it is useful in raising people's awareness of the need to change and in providing information on the impact of attempts to improve quality. The collection and provision of quantitative data on performance is one of the longest established approaches. In some countries it is referred to as audit (medical audit if just concerned with doctors' performance, otherwise clinical audit). Some countries, such as the USA, refer to 'utilization review'.

The information may be fed back passively or actively. Passive feedback means the data are simply disseminated and it is left to the recipients to decide what action to take. Active dissemination involves additional activities. For example, providing primary care doctors with information on their prescribing habits may be accompanied by a visit from a pharmaceutical adviser to discuss any atypical performance.

Incentives

Incentives come in several forms. First, they may either be financial (such as extra pay for carrying out an activity) or sociobehavioural, that is, appealing to workers' desire to be well regarded by their colleagues and peers. Second, incentives may be positive (rewarding good quality) or negative (penalizing poor quality).

Generally, professionals respond more to sociobehavioural incentives than financial ones, an observation that you should understand given what you have learned about the nature of professions in Chapter 6. Professionals set great store by what their peers think of them. Most people want to be respected within their own 'tribe'. Having said that, financial incentives can be effective in achieving some very specific change such as encouraging community health workers to increase immunization rates or the use of impregnated bed nets to prevent malaria. One of the most striking examples is the use of fixed payments for hospital admissions according to the patient's diagnosis (using some form of diagnosis-related groups). This acts as a disincentive to extend a patient's stay.

As regards positive versus negative incentives, people tend to respond more to positive promises than the fear of negative consequences.

Administrative structures and processes

One of the commonest reasons why poor quality care occurs is the way services are organized within a provider (health centre, community nursing service, hospital). While such problems may be manifest in numerous ways, there are four broad ways of reorganizing:

- change the availability of a service (e.g. introduce a list of essential drugs or a hospital formulary to avoid misuse);
- change access to a service (e.g. requests for diagnostic tests must specify the clinical justification or permit primary care doctors to request tests directly rather than having to refer the patient to a specialist first);
- change staff responsibilities (e.g. let nurses take over blood pressure checks from doctors);
- pre-authorization and concurrent review (e.g. a surgeon has to get permission from the purchaser of the service (such as a social insurance fund) before operating).

The scope for re-engineering (as it is sometimes called) the processes of health care is enormous. You have already learned about some of the options for staff substitution in Chapter 6. One of the attractions of these approaches is that the staff are often already well aware of the shortcomings of their service and have ideas as to how it could be improved. For example, if there are long delays for patients waiting in a clinic, the receptionist is more likely than the doctor to be the person to solve the problem. Involving staff in this way has the added benefit of their commitment and ownership of the solution.

You may be wondering in what way these options to improve quality differ from the general management of health services. The answer is that they don't. Quality improvement is part of the task of management. Managing the change of organization of services is a key option available to health services to improve quality.

Regulation

External regulation may be imposed in five main ways:

1 Financial payment – through contracts that specify the quality of care required.
2 Accreditation – this can apply to training programmes (e.g. determining whether or not a provider is a suitable place for training nurses); or to providing services (e.g. determining whether or not certain surgical operations can be performed). Accreditation tends to focus on the inputs available, such as staffing levels and equipment. Seeking accreditation is usually voluntary and, therefore, optional.
3 Certification – in some countries a provider has to obtain governmental approval before it can acquire particular equipment, usually expensive high tech kit.
4 Licensure – in most (perhaps all) countries, clinical staff are not allowed to practise unless they have been licensed to do so by a professional regulatory body. As you know from Chapter 6, this fulfils one of the characteristics of a profession, that of self-regulation.
5 Inspection – which may be regular and routine or reactive when a serious adverse event has occurred.

As regulation is both expensive and can antagonize those being regulated, these are approaches that should be used sparingly and only where it is essential (such as licensing professionals). The creation of resistance among the very people you hope to change may be counter-productive.

One danger of regulation is that those being regulated can gain control over the regulating body. A classic example is medical associations in which some members of the profession regulate their colleagues. This depends on the regulators remaining detached and avoiding being unduly influenced by the colleagues they are assessing. There is the danger of those being regulated defining the criteria by which they will be assessed. For example, surgeons may decide that they should be assessed solely in terms of their post-operative mortality, whereas patients might also want to see the surgeons' communication skills included.

Legislation

Behind all of these approaches lurks the threat of legal action being taken against individual staff or provider organizations if poor quality care occurs. The extent to which litigation occurs varies between countries depending on historical and cultural factors. There is a debate as to whether litigation (or the threat of it) helps improve the quality of care or harms it. Some argue that the fear of it leads providers to be 'defensive' and avoid taking risks. This may not be in a patient's interest. For example, it is argued that the high rates of Caesarean sections in some countries are because if an obstetrician perceives there might be any risk in leaving a woman to try and deliver vaginally, he or she will intervene and deliver the baby by Caesarean section. While such behaviour is understandable, it may be resulting in poorer quality care.

Quality improvement programmes

Whichever of the approaches described is adopted, quality improvement is more likely to be successful if:

- it has the support and involvement of the most respected opinion leaders in the area
- there is a sense of ownership by the participants
- participants recognize the need for change
- the focus is on improving quality rather than reducing costs
- a combination of approaches is used
- the methods used are changed every so often to ensure persistence of the change.

As with many aspects of health care, quality improvement has developed in high income countries. Some of the methods, such as the use of sophisticated computer-based methods, will clearly be inappropriate for low and middle income countries for some time. However, many methods can be used, albeit that some modification to more appropriate means need to be devised.

 Activity 20.3

The following paragraphs are extracts from an article by Willy De Geyndt (2001) in which he reviews the quality improvement programmes that have been initiated in four Latin American countries: Chile, Ecuador, Brazil and Argentina. As you read his account, note down the main factors that have affected the introduction of quality improvement. (Note that he refers to quality assurance (QA) rather than quality improvement.)

 Improving the quality of health care in Latin America

The evolution in Chile and Ecuador – two countries with similar population size (14.6 million and 12.5 million respectively) – shows an interesting contrast. External funding was the spark plug in both countries for initiating a quality assurance program. Outside funding in Chile ended 2 years and external technical assistance ended 4 years after start-up . . . Strong leadership in the Ministry of Health in Chile ensured allocation of its own resources in 1993 as well as the institutionalization of QA functions. QA activities were permanently incorporated in MOH's structure in 1995. Under the new title of 'Quality and Regulation Unit', the original focus on improving the quality of primary health care was broadened to measure the quality of all national health priorities. Indicators were developed to measure and improve the quality of 16 national health priorities. As implied by the unit's name, it also assessed the regulatory role of MOH in developing and promoting standards and monitoring compliance with standards.

External funding in Ecuador has been a major financing source of QA activities, and the contents and areas of application have been defined by mutual agreement between donors and the country. A ministerial decree 'institutionalized' a national QA program in 1996. By placing it in a parallel position to the MOH structure it was not incorporated into its formal organizational structure. Noteworthy is that both Chile and Ecuador 'institutional-ized' the QA programs but in one case it became an integral part of the organizational structure and in the other it was put on a parallel track. The well-intentioned proposals of the Ecuadorean government elected in 1998 had a slow start but advanced the agenda in three areas: (i) it included QA in the health sector reform program which emphasizes decentralization, with more autonomy for health service delivery units; (ii) the focus of QA expanded from primary health care, especially essential obstetric care (partly financed by USAID), to hospitals; and (iii) preliminary activities to develop hospital accreditation schemes were started. Following mass demonstrations in January 2000 a new government was installed with sector leadership less committed to QA and a slowing down of the initiatives of the previous 18-month-old government.

The lack of continuity and stability in sector leadership and the negative economic growth in Ecuador contrast sharply with Chile's record in institutionalizing, financing and expand-ing the scope of quality improvement efforts. Stable political leadership willing and able to make decisions is a key ingredient but so is availability and willingness to allocate resources to quality improvement programs . . .

Brazil started a national program in 1995 pulling together several initiatives that had started in the early 1990s [with] a 'Five Tracks Strategy':

• the use of outcomes indicators (mainly in pediatric and obstetric care);
• creating a national consortium for accrediting health care systems and services;
• developing selective quality improvement tools;
• producing clinical guidelines to decrease individual clinical practice variations;
• legislating consumer rights and protection (1990 law).

A larger number of approaches in Brazil may be justified as a better fit because of its population size (about 160 million), geographic size, cultural diversity and large socio-economic differences. Brazil has relied on a public/private sector mix to develop its QA programs. Two of the five tracks have been developed and promoted in the public sector: the use of outcomes indicators in maternal and childcare programs, and the consumer protection legislation. The government has been an active partner in developing accredit-ation standards, but a private sector consortium is the leading actor now. Clinical guide-lines are developed and used by medical societies. The use of quality improvement tools [quality prizes, quality awards and mentions, International Standards Organization (ISO) certification] is a mix of private and public initiatives.

Argentina and Brazil are using different methods and approaches. The hospital accredit-ation approach in Argentina focuses on structure. It measures the quality of inputs by determining the presence or absence of a large number of standards deemed critical to quality hospital care. The presence–absence model clearly reveals the absence of a stand-ard but hides the degree to which a standard is present – or should be present – and whether the standard is applied appropriately and consistently. Good quality of inputs – acceptable physical, financial, staffing and organizational structures – is conducive to good care but does not assure good care. They are necessary but not sufficient conditions. When followed up by intensive field surveys, the input data can also be used as a guide for inquiring into and assessing process and outcome dimensions of the care provided.

Brazil's approach is broader and encompasses the structure of care (accreditation, consumer protection), the process of providing care (clinical guidelines, quality improvement tools) and the results of providing the right inputs and using the correct process (outcome indicators). The report implies a vertically fragmented use of the structure, process and outcome measures. A weakness is not bringing to bear simultaneously the three elements of the widely accepted structure–process–outcome trilogy on the same health problems. Tackling health problems synergistically would yield superior results.

What can we learn from the experiences of Argentina, Brazil, Chile and Ecuador?

First, we need to acknowledge that the systematic and sustained use of quality assurance and quality improvement methods is in an early stage of introduction and development in Latin America with start-up and implementation in the 1990s.

Second, hospital accreditation seems to have developed and taken a stronger foothold in the two countries (Argentina and Brazil) that have a large private hospital sector.

Third, QA programs tend to be initiated and promoted by the public sector – often with external seed money financing – except for hospital accreditation where the private sector seems to assume the leadership. Medical schools, scientific societies and professional associations have been more involved in Argentina's national QA program than in the other three countries reviewed here.

Fourth, external funding by bilateral and multilateral agencies has helped in starting up and building support for QA programs; however, it is the allocation of a country's own resources that ensures expansion and institutionalization of the measurement and the continuous improvement of the quality of health care services.

Fifth, there seems to be a relationship between health sector leadership and especially continuity of leadership at the top and the allocation of internal financial resources for quality assurance and quality improvement programs.

Sixth, the incipient development and use of QA in Latin America merits support from the international QA community to ensure that quality assurance and improvement become permanent and sustainable parts of each country's health care delivery system.

 Feedback

The author identifies several factors that have contributed to successful implementation of quality improvement programmes:

- availability of external funding from donor countries
- availability of technical assistance from other countries
- strong and stable leadership in the Ministry of Health
- incorporation of the programme in the main organizational structure rather than letting it run in parallel
- commitment of the country's own funds after an initial period of external assistance rather than a reliance on donors
- involvement both of the public and the private sector (in countries where both exist)
- involvement of professional associations in collaboration with government initiatives.

Summary

In most countries a variety of approaches to quality improvement are being used. It is important to ensure that such diverse activities complement each other and that providers and the public are not confused and, even worse, antagonized. You have seen how activities can be mapped in terms of their location (internal or external) and their timing (reactive or proactive). You have learned about the six main forms of intervention to improve quality, and the need to use combinations of approaches for the maximum impact.

References

Black N (1990). Quality assurance in medical care. *Journal of Public Health Medicine* 12: 97–104.
De Geyndt W (2001). Improving the quality of health care in Latin America. *International Journal of Quality in Health Care* 13: 85–7.

Glossary

Accreditation A voluntary survey of quality standards, performed by an independent body awarding grades.

Allocative (Pareto, social) efficiency A situation in which it is not possible to improve the welfare of one person in an economy without making someone else worse off.

Ambulatory care Health care provided to patients without admitting them to hospital, such as general practice, outpatient clinics and day care.

Appropriateness A health care intervention is deemed appropriate if the benefits that result outweigh the costs (all aspects, not just financial) by a sufficiently wide amount.

Audit Review of performance usually judged against agreed criteria and standards.

Bamako Initiative An international initiative in 1987 based on primary health care principles with focus on community financing and decentralization.

Burden of disease A measure of the physical, emotional, social and financial impact that a particular disease has on the health and functioning of the population.

Bureaucracy A formal type of organization involving hierarchy, impersonality, continuity and expertise.

Capitation payments A prospective means of paying health care staff based on the number of people they provide care for.

Case series Study of a series of cases to identify common or recurring features.

Case study Observation and analysis of a single case to generate a hypothesis.

Case mix The mix of cases (or patients) that a provider cares for.

CATWOE a mnemonic for 'customers, actors, transformation, *Weltanschauung*, ownership and environment'.

Clinical guidelines Advice based on the best available research evidence and clinical experience.

Clinical or professional judgement The decision taken by a clinician as to whether or not a patient has a normative need.

Community financing Collective action of local communities to finance health services through pooling out-of-pocket payments and ensuring services are accountable to the community.

Community participation A process by which individuals or groups assume responsibility for health matters of their community.

Compliance The extent to which a patient follows professional advice.

Comprehensive primary care A comprehensive health strategy (outlined in the Alma-Ata Declaration) based on equity, a multisectoral approach, community participation, appropriate technologies, and health promotion.

Consensus development A set of explicit formal methods for developing and establishing the collective views of a group when faced with uncertainty.

Consumerism A social movement promoting and representing user interests in health services.

Co-payments (user fees) Direct payments made by users of health services as a contribution to their cost (e.g. prescription charges).

Corporate rationalizers A contemporary approach to management in which the organization (corporation) attempts to dominate professional autonomy through the use of measurement and data.

Cross-boundary flow The use of services by people who are not resident in the local area of the facility.

Culture The values, beliefs and attitudes associated with a social system.

Decentralization The transfer of authority and responsibility from central government to local levels, which are thereby strengthened.

Demand Expressed need for health services.

Disability (also referred to as functional status) The impact on the patient's ability to function.

Disability-adjusted life years (DALYs) A measure of health based not only on the length of a person's life but also their level of ability (or disability).

Discourse The way language is used in a particular area of social life.

Disease A condition which, judged by the prevailing culture, is painful or disabling and deviates from either the statistical norm or from some idealized status.

Diseases Patterns of factors (symptoms, signs) that occur in many people in more or less the same way.

Disease-specific measures Instruments that focus on the particular aspects of the disease being studied.

Empathy A response that demonstrates understanding and acceptance of the patient's feelings and concerns.

Encounter The interaction of two or more people in a face-to-face meeting.

Environmental turbulence The ever changing external pressures on an organization and its managers such as legislation, the national economy, professional associations and trades unions, and public opinion.

Essential package of care A strategy for purchasing services that achieves the greatest reduction in the burden of disease with available resources.

Fee-for-service A means of paying health care staff on the basis of the actual items of care provided.

Felt need A person's subjective assessment of their need for better health.

Formal care Care provided by trained, paid professionals, usually in a formal setting.

Generic measures Instruments that measure general aspects of a person's health, such as mobility, sleeping and appetite.

Gross domestic product (GDP) The market value of the goods and services produced within the borders of a country (consumption plus investment plus government purchases plus net exports).

Gross national product (GNP) The market value of the goods and services produced by the nationals of a country irrespective of where they reside (i.e. includes expatriates and excludes resident foreigners).

Health services research (HSR) A multidisciplinary activity to improve the quality, organization and management of health services. HSR is not itself a discipline.

Holism The conceptualization of a system as a whole and the belief that the whole is greater than the sum of the parts.

Horizontal equity The equal treatment of individuals or groups in the same circumstances.

Horizontal programmes Health services organized to provide care across a range of diseases at one level (usually primary care).

Iatrogenesis Disease resulting from medical or health care interventions.

Ideal type A hypothetical model of a complex real phenomenon which emphasizes its most salient features.

Ideology A set of beliefs, values and attitudes used to justify and legitimize power.

Illness behaviour The way a person behaves when they feel a need for better health.

Impairment The physical signs of the condition (pathology), usually measured by clinicians.

Inputs The resources needed by a system.

Intermediate care Residential or inpatient care for those who have been in hospital but are not yet ready to go home and for those who need inpatient care but are not so ill as to require the services of a major hospital.

Inverse care law The observation that availability of care appears to be inversely related to need.

Lay care Care provided by lay people who have received no formal training and are not paid. It includes self-care, care by relatives, friends and self-help groups.

Length of stay The length of time a patient stays in hospital.

Litigation Legal action taken by patients against health care providers for alleged malpractice.

Macroeconomic efficiency The total costs of the health system in relation to overall health status. Countries differ in how efficiently their health systems convert resources used into health gains.

Medical cosmology The study of medical paradigms.

Medicalization The tendency of doctors increasingly to define areas as being 'medical' and thus subject to their influence and control in the belief that this is helpful (also referred to as medical imperialism).

Medical paradigm The prevailing thoughts and knowledge about health and disease.

Meta-analysis An overview of all the valid research evidence. If feasible, the quantitative results of different studies may be combined to obtain an overall result, referred to as a 'statistical meta-analysis'.

Microeconomic efficiency The scope for achieving greater efficiency from existing resources. It is of two types – allocative and technical efficiency.

Multidimensional model An analytical approach integrating selected socio-economic, cultural and organizational factors.

Normative need A professional assessment of a person's need for health care based on objective measures.

Not-for-profit organizations Organization with no shareholders, so all income received for providing services is paid to staff or invested in improving the organization.

Outcomes Change in status as a result of the system processes (in the health services context, the change in health status as a result of care).

Outputs A combination of the processes and outcomes that constitute the total production of a system.

Pathological Relating to form or function that is deemed to be abnormal.

Payers (funders) The people who provide funds to pay for health care. In a tax-based system, the tax payers; in a social insurance system, employees and employers.

Physiological Relating to bodily function (such as breathing) that is deemed to be 'normal'.

Power The ability to influence, and in particular to control, resources.

Primary care Formal care that is the first point of contact for people. It is usually general rather than specialized, and provided in the community.

Processes The use of resources or the activity within a system.

Profession An occupation based on specified knowledge and training and regulated standards of performance.

Professional autonomy The freedom that professionals have to make decisions without being accountable to their employers or the state.

Professionalization A process whereby an occupation achieves the more independent status of a profession.

Prospective payment Paying providers before any care is delivered, based on predefined activity levels and anticipated costs.

Providers Organizations (hospitals, health centres) or individuals (community nurses) who provide care.

Purchasers Those who purchase health services from providers on behalf of those eligible to use health care. In public systems this may be government or public bodies; in social insurance systems, the insurance company or sick fund.

Quality criteria Statements that describe what constitutes good quality care.

Quality improvement A systematic approach to assessing, monitoring and improving the performance of health services according to defined standards.

Quality of care The extent to which care is effective, humane and equitable.

Quality of life (handicap or well-being) The impact of the condition on the social functioning of a person, partly determined by the person's environment.

Quality standards The desired level of compliance with a quality criterion.

Random variation Statistical differences that occur by chance and are inevitable when counting events.

Reductionism Consideration of the component parts rather than the whole organism or organization.

Relative need Comparison between needs of individuals with similar conditions or between needs of populations living in similar areas.

Reliability The extent to which an instrument produces consistent results.

Responsiveness The extent to which an instrument detects real changes in the state of health of a person.

Retrospective payment Paying providers for any work they have undertaken, with no agreement in advance.

Risk (case-mix) adjustment A statistical process to make allowance for any difference in case mix between providers when comparing their performance.

Root definition A description of a system based on each of the elements of CATWOE.

Secondary care Specialized care that often can only be accessed by being referred by a primary care worker. It is usually provided in local hospitals.

Selective primary care An interim strategy until comprehensive primary care is available for all, based on selection of cost-effective medical interventions.

Self-help groups Groups of unpaid, self-taught people who offer solutions to health problems in a lay setting, based on mutual support between persons experiencing similar conditions.

Sickness (sick) funds Non-governmental purchasing organisations in social insurance schemes.

Skills mix The mix of posts, grades or occupations in an organization. It may also refer to the combinations of activities or skills needed for each job within the organization.

Social role A set of ideas and actions that let individuals behave according to expected social norms.

Standardized mortality ratio (SMR) An indicator of the frequency of deaths in a population that takes into account the age and sex structure of the population.

Substitution A process replacing existing services with more appropriate ones, through changes in location of care, technology, and staff and skills mix.

Syndicalism A militant trade union movement aimed at transferring the control and ownership of the means of production to unions.

System A model of a whole entity, reflecting the relationship between its elements at different levels of complexity.

Systematic review A review of the literature that uses an explicit approach to searching, selecting and combining the relevant studies.

Systematic variation Statistical differences that cannot be accounted for by the inevitable random variations that occur when counting events.

Technical (operational, productive) efficiency Using only the minimum necessary resources to finance, purchase and deliver a particular activity or set of activities (i.e. avoiding waste).

Tertiary care Highly specialized care that often can only be accessed by referral from secondary care. It is usually proved in national or regional hospitals.

Total quality management (continuous quality improvement) An approach to quality improvement that involves the commitment of all members of an organization to meeting the needs of its external and internal customers.

Use Utilization of health services that are actually provided.

Utilization rate A measurement of health service use.

Validity The extent to which an instrument measures what it intends to measure.

Vertical equity The principle that individuals who are unequal should be treated differently according to their level of need.

Vertical programmes Health services focused on a single disease or population group (such as children) encompassing all levels of care.

Index